Caring and Communicating

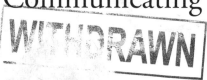

Related titles from Macmillan

Paul Morrison and Philip Burnard
Caring and Communicating: Facilitator's Manual
Second Edition

Philip Burnard and Paul Morrison
Nursing Research in Action
Second Edition

CARING AND COMMUNICATING
The Interpersonal Relationship in Nursing

Second Edition

PAUL MORRISON

Associate Professor – School of Nursing
Queensland University of Technology

PHILIP BURNARD

Vice Dean of the School of Nursing Studies
University of Wales College of Medicine

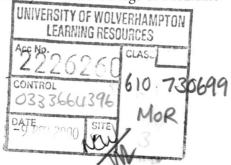

MACMILLAN

Published by
MACMILLAN PRESS LTD
Houndmills, Basingstoke, Hampshire RG21 6XS
and London
Companies and representatives
throughout the world

ISBN 0–333–66439–6 paperback

A catalogue record for this book is available
from the British Library.

This book is printed on paper suitable for recycling and made from fully managed and sustained forest sources.

10 9   8   7   6   5   4   3   2
06 05 04 03 02 01 00

Editing and origination by
Aardvark Editorial, Mendham, Suffolk

Printed in China

First edition 1991
Reprinted 1992, 1993, 1995
Second edition 1997

For Jim, Kathleen, Franziska, Sarah and Maeve
and for Sally, Aaron and Rebecca

Contents

Acknowledgement

Thanks are due to Baillière Tindall for permission to
reproduce a shortened account of some material that appeared in
Morrison, P (1994) *Understanding Patients.*

Introduction

The interpersonal relationship in nursing

Since the publication of the first edition of this book, many things in nursing have changed. We have seen an increased interest in the study of *caring* as a component of nursing. We have also seen interpersonal and communication skills training become part of mainstream nursing education. That education has also moved into higher education, and more attention has been paid to grounding nursing in research. Our aim in preparing this new edition is to offer more evidence of some of these changes – theoretical, practical and research-based. We have also offered a more *critical* account of the ideas contained in the first edition and feel that this is appropriate.

This book is about caring and communicating in nursing – in all branches of the profession, from community care to adult nursing, and from mental health nursing to care of the child. Its aim is to help diploma, undergraduate and postgraduate students to explore their interpersonal relationships with patients and colleagues. Now that nursing has moved into higher education, it is important that nurses combine practical and interpersonal skills with research findings and reports from the literature. We offer some examples of the studies in caring and communicating that we have been involved in over the past 10 years. In these examples, we explore some methodological and substantive issues. The research will show how different methods often lead to different types of result or finding. The findings presented are laid out in different ways. These should give the reader an insight into some approaches to research in this area.

■ Change in nursing

Nursing has changed. New theories, new models of nursing flourish and new educational methods have brought new skills to the community and hospital clinical setting. We have also seen a greater emphasis placed on *primary care* and on the nurse working closely with other health professionals in the 'front line' of care. The patient-centred philosophies of recent years have brought with them the need for nurses to reconsider how they plan and carry out the process of nursing. Within all this change, however, two aspects of nursing have remained constant: the need to *care* and the need to *communicate*. Both are essential aspects of the process of nursing. Both, too, are recognised in the new educational programmes being developed in nursing that look towards the year 2000.

The concepts of caring and communicating have not remained static. What may have been considered 'caring' in the past may not correspond to how we perceive caring today. Just as styles of nursing have changed, so have approaches to caring. However, it is still not clear what we mean when we use the term 'caring relationship' in nursing.

Communication, in the past, tended to be a 'top down' and chain-like affair, doctors communicating with senior ward staff, senior ward staff with junior ward staff, and so on. Communication with patients was often (and perhaps still is) a hit and miss activity: the patient often had little or no clear idea about what was happening to him or her. In recent years, we have seen a rapid growth in all aspects of communication in nursing. Nursing curricula have included interpersonal skills and counselling as essential topics to be covered. Management and clinical staff are attending assertiveness courses, self-awareness workshops and courses on counselling. Most nurses are becoming more aware of the need to communicate effectively with all of the people with whom they have contact. *Poor* communication is one of the factors that encourages most complaints about professional care. We must learn to communicate more effectively.

■ Developments in the nurse–patient relationship

Perhaps the most marked changes in nursing have come about in the relationship that exists between nurses and patients. Patients are no longer passive recipients of care, just as student nurses are no longer passive recipients of nursing education (although the latter situation is taking longer to change than the former). People who come into hospital or who are cared for in their homes are now better informed about health care, are becoming more likely to question their care and are rightly demanding a higher standard of health care.

Several reasons for this change could be suggested: television programmes and advertisements on health-related issues are now common-
place; Sunday newspaper supplements often run articles on changes in
health provision; educational programmes in schools and colleges are
encouraging people to be more aware of their health needs and more questioning of the care they receive; and nurses and doctors are generally being
called to account not only for what they do but also for why they do it.
The Patients' Charter has also made all health care professionals more
aware of the need to monitor their own performance – although responses
to the Patients' Charter have been mixed. The 'named nurse' feature of the
Charter has, however, meant that nurses have become more focused in
their work and clearer about what their obligations are to their patients.

The traditional roles of doctors and nurses are changing, and that
change is forcing nurses to reappraise the way they deliver care and the
way in which they communicate with their patients and colleagues.
Also, nurses, doctors and other health care professionals are, increasingly, being *taught* together, and this is likely to make all of the professional disciplines more aware of each group's problems and strengths.
Interdisciplinary teaching has the potential to promote greater teamwork among professionals and begin to break down professional
communication barriers.

These issues raise many questions: What generalisations can be made
about caring? Can caring be taught? What aspects of communication in
nursing need most attention? How can nurses improve their communication skills? More specifically, it may be useful if you stop at this point and
consider the following questions for yourself:

- What do I mean when I use the word 'caring'?
- In what situations do I consider myself 'caring' and in what situations
  am I less than caring?
- How did I learn to care?
- How do I monitor my caring?
- What are the problems I encounter in caring for others?
- In what ways do I communicate with others?
- What are my best means of communicating?
- In what ways do my communicating skills need enhancing?
- How did I learn to communicate?
- What are the most frequent problems I have when trying to
  communicate?

These questions and many others of a similar nature are addressed
directly in this book. In the following pages, we outline a provisional
theory that draws together the process of caring and the process of
communicating as they influence the work of the nurse. Evidence from

the literature and from current research about aspects of caring and communicating is reported and discussed. We believe that both caring and communication skills can be enhanced and developed in all nurses. To that end, we offer practical suggestions about training and further research.

The figure below provides a simple model that acts as a guideline for understanding the content of the book. In the model, we note that the two concepts of caring and communicating arise as the two most important and constant aspects of nursing. The two concepts involve overlapping (although sometimes different) knowledge, skills and attitudes. The person who is able to develop some knowledge, skills and attitudes is able to develop 'a caring relationship' with others. This, in turn, has a positive effect on all those people with whom the nurse comes into contact: patients, relatives, colleagues, family, friends and others.

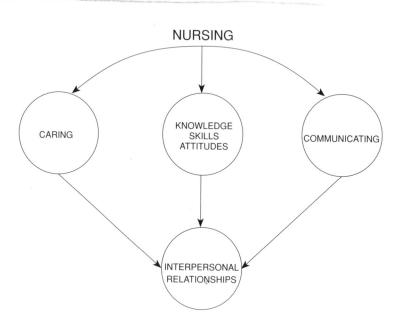

A simple model of caring and communicating in
interpersonal relationships in nursing

The point of such a model is not to explain in great detail all the aspects involved in caring and communicating. Instead, the aim is to offer a description and a starting point for the more formal study of these two domains. Through the use of the model, it will be possible, later in the book, to show some of the implications of the knowledge and research contained in it for day-to-day practice, for education and training, and for further research.

It is worth reflecting for a moment on your own education. Did it contain a thorough introduction to aspects of communicating with others? Did you learn a range of usable interpersonal skills? What did you learn about caring? Did you learn *how* to care? Or was it assumed that you knew how? After all, people become nurses because they want to care for other people and to help, and everybody knows what this process entails!

It is asserted here that many nurses have to date received only a very basic introduction to communication training and very little training in the domain of caring. It is with these factors in mind that we have tried to formalise some of the aspects of caring and communicating in the above model. Both caring and communicating are complex phenomena. It is only through attempting to break them down into manageable components that we can begin to work with them. As nursing progresses towards the year 2000, it is essential that nurses develop caring and communication skills in both hospital and community settings. Many of the new nursing programmes are geared towards equipping nurses with these essential skills.

The book, then, is an analysis of the theory and practice of caring and communicating, offering reports from recent research and theory from the literature to enable you to explore your own caring and communication skills in nursing practice. We hope, too, that the book will lead to the enhancement of what is perhaps best described as the 'caring relationship': the relationship that enables us to both care and communicate with our patients, in whatever field of nursing we work.

■ Layout of the book

This book is divided in two distinct but interrelated parts. Part One, 'Caring and Nursing', examines some of the theoretical notions and research-based findings in studies into what it means to care for another person and how care is experienced by the recipient. The essential link between the work of the nurse and the process of caring for another person is emphasised. In Part Two, 'Communicating and Nursing', we explore theory and research findings related to the role of communication skills in the practice of nursing care. A number of theoretical frameworks are examined, which may provide opportunities for further research in this difficult and demanding domain. We also describe some of the theory and report research findings focusing directly on nurse education. We advocate the 'experiential learning' format as the one of choice in teaching and learning caring and communication skills. These skills are the key to competent nursing practice.

Finally, we hope that you find the book useful. It is not intended to be an exhaustive analysis of the two topics, nor is it supposed to be merely a list of prescriptions. We hope that you will try out what we suggest and that you will read the book critically. We are all fairly skilled at avoiding doing anything about our lives: if anything is to change in terms of our nursing care, we have to modify our behaviour, we have to try out new things. We hope that this book will spark off ideas about how you can make small changes and experiment with your presentation of self and with your approach to nursing.

Paul Morrison
Associate Professor – School of Nursing
Queensland University of Technology
Kelvin Grove Campus
Brisbane
Australia

Philip Burnard
Vice Dean of the School of Nursing Studies
University of Wales College of Medicine
Heath Park
Cardiff
UK

PART ONE

Caring and Nursing

Chapter One

What is caring?

We work in a caring profession. Yet what do we mean by 'caring'? In a common-sense sort of way, we all know what it feels like to feel cared for or to care for another person. At another level, however, the issue becomes more complicated. Can we, for instance, say that we all mean the same thing when we use the word 'caring'? Is the caring that you experience in a relationship within the family the same as that which you experience when caring for a patient? Probably not.

In this chapter, we explore the notion of caring by considering how various writers have defined caring. It may be useful if you consider what they have to say and compare *their* definitions and descriptions of caring with your own. We explore a general analysis of the concept of caring as well as a specific view of caring as it relates to nursing. Later, in other chapters, we will consider the research that has been undertaken in this field.

■ The phenomenon of caring

Milton Mayeroff, in an analysis of the meaning of caring in human relationships (Mayeroff, 1972), describes caring as a process that offers people (both carers and cared-for) opportunities for personal growth. Major aspects of caring in the analysis include:

- knowledge
- alternating rhythms (learning from experience)
- patience
- honesty
- trust
- humility
- hope, and
- courage.

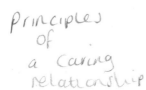

principles of a caring relationship

The general theme in this account is that caring can influence people's lives in a significant way and lead to a more fulfilled existence. What we find in Mayeroff's account are broad principles of caring. The problem is that they may not be specific enough to apply to all caring situations. You may not agree that they are the *necessary* components of caring at all. It may be useful, at this point, to stop and jot down your own list of criteria for what are the main ingredients of a caring relationship and to compare them with the list above.

Mayeroff is concerned with caring in the most general sense. His analysis was not meant to be confined to caring in a clinical or health care setting. Mayeroff was concerned with *all* caring relationships: personal, interpersonal, familial, spiritual, therapeutic, emotional, and so on. It may be useful, now, to turn to a more applied analysis of caring as offered by Alistair Campbell.

Campbell (1984a) has discussed the curious notion of health professionals being paid to care for others. It is, indeed, possible to question whether or not care can be prescribed or carried out as an intentional, professional act. It seems likely that the professional caring relationship is different from other caring relationships, if only in the sense that in a professional caring relationship we do not have the degree of *choice* about caring that exists in most other day-to-day relationships.

The concept of 'skilled companionship' (Campbell, 1984a) may be preferable to that of 'carer' as a description of the relationship that exists between the paid health professional and his or her patient. Companionship, says Campbell, may be differentiated by the characteristics described below.

❏ Closeness without sexual stereotyping

Companionship, unlike caring, is usually devoid of a sexual connotation. I may be a companion to a person to whom I am not sexually attracted and who does not necessarily find me so. Companionship, also, does not raise issues of heterosexuality and homosexuality. It is usually quite acceptable for men to have male companions and women female companions. While this may sometimes be true in the caring situation, the concept of caring is perhaps a more intimate one. The notion of companionship seems to circumnavigate these social, sexual issues. Also, and perhaps more contentiously, the idea of romantic love is less likely to be an issue in companionship than in caring.

❏ Movement and change

Companionship, because it is less intense than a full caring relationship, is more open to movement and change. As the carer and the one being cared for are less dependent on each other than is the case in a caring relationship, each party can develop and grow at his or her own rate. Campbell suggests that:

> The good companion is someone who shares freely, but does not impose, allowing others to make their *own* journey. (Campbell, 1984a)

Perhaps, for some, the companionship relationship is less claustrophobic than the caring relationship.

[handwritten: Nurse and other members are companion]

The other point about movement is that the companion is the person who 'travels with' the other person, who assists, encourages and supports the other to recovery or death. The concept of movement is totally absent in those forms of institutional care where the prevailing norms are stasis, unchanging routine, resigned acceptance and lack of hope. So then, is the concept of companionship lost in these circumstances?

❏ Mutuality

Companionship suggests mutuality. In accompanying another person, we share the relationship, and each supports and helps the other. The *degree* to which this is possible in the nursing field is a matter of some contention. Carl Rogers, discussing therapeutic relationships, suggests that the relationship between the one being helped and the helper *is* a mutual one. The philosopher Martin Buber (1966) disagreed with Rogers and suggested that, because it is always the patient who comes to the professional for help and not the other way round, the relationship can never be a mutual one.

[handwritten: Look up mutual.]

❏ Commitment with defined limits

The companion, unlike the lover, is in an interesting situation regarding commitment. Campbell points out that companionship is less than friendship, yet it does require that the companion is prepared to invest time and energy in the relationship. The main difference, perhaps, between the relationship with lovers and friends and that with companions and those being accompanied is the fact that the companionship relationship exists within certain limits. In a friendship, those limits are worked out, informally and tacitly. Often friends do not try to define the limits of their relationship. The same can be said of the relationship between lovers.

On the other hand, the companion in the health care setting works within a specified code of conduct which offers the broadest outline for the relationship. The relationship is then further delineated by nurses' 'informal' concept of what is professional. In other words, most nurses have a picture, passed on from working with colleagues, of what is and what is not acceptable in a relationship with patients. This limiting of the relationship makes it different in an important way from other types of close relationship.

The other constraint on the companionship relationship in nursing is the fact that nurses work to time. They work shifts and see the people they care for for limited periods and at prearranged times. Also, nurses have to make decisions about how *much* time they can spend with particular patients. If, as is usually the case, they have responsibility for more than one person, it is likely that they will have to make decisions about how best to allocate their time to various people. While friends obviously have to consider how they use their time, the time factor is usually of less importance. In the case of lovers, time becomes important again, but in the opposite direction: lovers tend to want to spend as *much* time with each other as is possible.

While friendships may also be limited by time, the constraints are usually less formal. Friends normally *choose* the times that they meet, whereas nurses may be prescribed times for meeting the people for whom they care. Campbell's suggestion, then, is that the term 'skilled companionship' avoids some of the problems associated with caring in nursing and is a more fitting descriptor of the type of caring (or even loving) relationship that occurs between a nurse and her patients.

❏ The relationship between nursing and caring

Several authors have referred to caring in nursing as a form of loving. Ray (1981a) found that:

> a conceptual analysis of caring from different perspectives is suggestive of a form of loving...

While Campbell's (1984a) theological analysis of professional care, as we suggested above, required that caring be perceived as a form of 'moderated love'. The notion of moderated love suggests, as we have seen, that professional caring relationships are carefully bounded (or 'moderated') both by convention and by statute.

However, McFarlane (1976) referred to nursing as the process of 'helping, assisting, serving, caring', suggesting that nursing and caring were inseparable and at the same time indicating that some practical activities were involved in the caring process in nursing settings. This point of view was taken up and expanded on by Griffin (1980, 1983), who divided up the concept of caring into two major domains. One of these deals with nurses' attitudes and emotions, while the other is concerned with the activities the nurse engages in while carrying out her nursing function.

Interpersonal relationship

Griffin (1983) describes caring in nursing as essentially an interpersonal process, in which the nurse is required to carry out specific role-related activities in a way that conveys to the recipient the expression of certain emotions. The activities Griffin has in mind include assisting, helping and serving the person who has special needs. This process is influenced by the relationship which the nurse has with the patient. The emotions of 'liking' and 'compassion' were offered tentatively as important affective responses which are expressed through this relationship. Other aspects of attitude are discussed in later chapters.

While this analysis is useful, in that it suggests points of focus for those interested in the concept of caring, it fails to provide the type and depth of understanding required of a profession who claim caring as their central theme. In addition, this type of philosophical analysis has the disadvantage of being far removed from the practice of nursing and is likely to omit relevant considerations.

The centrality of caring to nursing has been widely affirmed (McFarlane, 1976; Watson, 1979, 1985; Leininger, 1981a). The Briggs Report claimed that nursing was *the* major caring profession. Indeed, Chapman (1983) suggested that one of the main reasons why people enter nursing was their desire to help and care for others at their most needy. Pratt (1980) similarly argued that caring was a major driving force for motivating people to enter the profession of nursing. Along similar lines, a specific selection interview has been developed for identifying candidates most likely to be successful in their nursing careers (Selection Research Limited, 1987). Caring was one of the 11 attributes isolated as likely predictors of success.

The influence of caring may also be demonstrated in its potential for determining acceptable and desirable levels of nursing care in practice situations (Carper, 1979; Kitson, 1987). Carper (1979) notes that 'caring as a *definition of caring* professional and personal value, is of central importance in providing a normative standard which governs our action and our attitudes toward those for whom we care' (pp. 11–12). In health care education generally, caring is a key concept (Bendall, 1977; Sarason, 1985), but it is perhaps ironic that a concept of such importance to nursing has received so little empirical attention from nurse researchers (Partridge, 1978; Leininger, 1981a, b). Commenting on the dearth of research in the area, Leininger (1981b) remarked:

Therapeutic tool.

The relationship between caregivers and care recipients is limitedly known, and yet this relationship appears to be the heart of therapeutic help to clients.

In effect we are left with a number of ideas about the nature of caring and caring relationships. Do we accept these views and opinions at face value? If so, can we put them to any practical use? The answer on both counts has to be no. For if caring is really so important to nursing, we must set out to explore systematically the process in great detail and be able to describe fully the nurse's caring role. To do this we need research methods and techniques suited to the task.

■ Why should nurses care?

This question can be addressed in several ways, but there are three important aspects that underpin the nurse's need to care for other people. These are the *contractual* aspect, the *ethical* aspect and the *spiritual* aspect of caring for others who are ill. Summarising these points and highlighting their ethical position, Fry (1988) suggests the following pointers about caring:

* Caring must be viewed as an ultimate or overriding value to guide one's actions.
* Caring must be considered a universal value.
* Caring must be considered prescriptive in that certain behaviours (empathy, support, compassion, protection, etc.) are preferred.
* Caring must be other-regarding – it must consider the human flourishing of others' and not one's own welfare.

❏ The contractual aspect

It has to be acknowledged that, as professionals, we are under a contractual obligation to care. As Radsma (1994) notes, 'nurses have a professional mandate to provide care'. It could be argued that being a nurse involves the notion of caring and that to offer clients a nursing service is to offer them care. Not to offer them care, on the other hand, is not to offer them nursing. In this sense, nursing is *defined* in relation to care. To nurse, then, is to care.

At a more concrete level, it might be argued that care is offered on the basis of patient or consumer expectation. We might say that the patient or client *expects* care from a nurse as part of the contract into which they have entered. To be a patient, in this case, is to expect care, and to be a nurse, in this case, is to offer that care. Nurses are also *employed* to offer care. Here, the nature of the contract between nurses and employees is based on an expectation that nurses will offer care. It needs to be said, however, that such a contractual issue is more an *implicit* than an explicit one.

If caring *is* a contractual issue, we need to consider the implications of this. Campbell (1984a) notes the apparent contradiction in the professional carer's role – health professionals are called upon to care but are also *paid* to do so. It is as though health professionals are, according to their financial contract, being called upon to 'turn on' their care. A similar state of affairs is found in counselling and psychotherapy, in which the client pays a professional person to sympathise, empathise and listen. The open question remains: can a person care both *professionally* and for money?

The sort of debate that usually occurs at this point is whether or not a paid carer is 'genuine'. The argument seems to revolve around the idea that genuiness is somehow a 'natural' state of affairs, whereas the introduction of a profit motive brings an unnaturalness to the proceedings. This sort of argument often surfaces when people discuss the naturalness or otherwise of those who work in service industries – hotels, restaurants, fast food facilities or flight attendants on aircraft. It has been suggested that if people have to be *trained* to work with the public, they are likely to be 'artificial' or 'unnatural'.

However, it could be argued that we have *all* 'learned' to relate to others in different contexts. If we care, we do so because we have *learned* to care and because it is an appropriate response in that context. That learning process may have occurred over a number of years. It might be argued, for example, that we learned to care by being cared for – by parents, friends, lovers and partners. We have experienced care and are therefore able to show care in return. We may also have learned to care vicariously – by observing other people being cared for. All of this amounts to a learning process.

If we return to the debate about professional carers, we may find that cabin crew, hotel staff, and so on have also *learned* to care – but have done so in a highly structured, intentional way. The process has been speeded up and, although the *methods of learning* may be different, it can still be argued that such staff have learned to care. So may it be with nurses. There is no reason why we should automatically assume that caring 'comes naturally' to some people, nor even that it must always be spontaneous and straight from the heart.

There is another element to the *contractual* aspect of caring. Homans (1961) proposed a theory of social exchange when he suggested that:

> The open secret of human exchange is to give to the other person behaviour that is more valuable to him than it is costly to you and to get from him behaviour that is more valuable to you than it is costly to him.

For Homans, interpersonal life is a series of transactions in which each person does things for and with another person in anticipation of receiving something. This is a day-to-day example of the general rule that people usually 'give and take' in their relationships with others in a mutually agreed fashion. In this context, it means that nurses care in order to get something in return – perhaps job satisfaction, the sense of achievement, contact with people and a salary at the end of the month. All these things can make the job rewarding and worthwhile, and encourage us to invest something of ourselves in it.

Another facet of the contractual aspect may be found in the writing of Martin Buber (1958), who compared and contrasted the 'I–It' personal relationship with the 'I–Thou' personal relationship. In essence, Buber's contention was this: that when we deal with people on an 'I–It' basis, we turn those people into objects. This sort of objectification can be seen when we refer to other people as 'the appendix in bed six' and has the effect of turning a living person into 'an appendix' – an object. Buber argues that a more human – and more morally defensible position – is to treat people from the point of view of an 'I–Thou' relationship. In such a relationship, each person meets the other as a conscious, knowing and feeling human being who is respected.

Buber is arguing that an essential part of the process of working with other human beings is to acknowledge *their* humanness. Part of the 'contract' of being a carer or a therapist is *not* to turn them into an object but to allow them to remain not only people, but also people on equal terms with ourselves. This can only be achieved through constant vigilance and a great deal of humility. If we are to retain the 'I–Thou' mode of relations, we must forego any 'professional' pretensions that we may have. For to treat people from a professional point of view might involve turning them into objects.

These are just some of the issues that influence the contractual aspect of professional care. Nurse–patient relationships may be seen as variously defined and negotiated relationships that involve some sort of give and take on behalf of the two participants. In such relationships, each participant is seen as having some sort of need. The professional nurse takes on a contract to care.

❏ The ethical aspect

Ethical questions are questions of right or wrong, of how to make appropriate decisions, of how to act in a given situation. These sorts of question will affect the way a nurse cares. There are various ways of approaching ethical issues. A religious code of some sort that instructs the believer in ways to act could be evoked. Indeed, it should be noted that most religious codes urge believers to act caringly towards other people. We might even be tempted to argue that a religious person is usually duty bound to act in a caring way towards others. Ironically, however, we also know that religion is also behind many of the international instances of people not caring for each other – ethnic cleansing, genocide and wars often have links with extreme religious beliefs.

We need, then, to turn to secular approaches to the ethics of caring. By secular, we mean those approaches that do not draw on religious codes of behaviour – although the two are often compatible. There is no reason to suppose that a secular approach to ethics automatically rules out a particular religious code.

A widely cited source of guidance in ethical matters is Kant's injunction that we should act as though our behaviour were illustrating a universal law of behaviour. In other words, when we act, we must do so believing that the behaviour would be one in which *anyone* might reasonably engage. A right action, then, is one that is *universally* right. This is the basis of Kant's *categorical imperative*. It is possible to argue from this position that the reason we *should* care is that we would hope to be cared for ourselves. We would also hope that care would be extended to all the people whom we know and love. In this way, caring is almost a necessary human behaviour because an *absence* of care is, by the same token, unacceptable as a universal principle. Presumably, we would not want to live in a world in which no-one cared for others, so caring becomes an imperative.

Another approach to considering the ethical rationale for caring is Mill's *utilitarianism* – an approach first articulated by Jeremy Bentham. Utilitarianism is often summed up by the slogan, or slight variants of it, that 'that which is good is that which causes the greatest happiness to the greatest number'. It seems reasonable to argue that caring is *unlikely* to cause widespread unhappiness and it can, therefore, be justified as a 'good' action. A more positive perspective suggests that caring *will* cause fairly widespread happiness and can, again, be justified. All this, of course, hangs on how 'caring' might be defined and this, again, has been the subject of debate throughout this volume. It would be hard, however, to argue that caring was *not* a 'positive' concept.

Yet another approach to ethics is through *existentialism*. Existentialism is a particular and distinctive approach to philosophy. The most populist definition of existentialism as an approach to philosophy was offered by Jean-Paul Sartre in his 1949 essay *Existentialism and Humanism* (Sartre, 1952). Sartre sums up the heart of existentialism through the slogan 'existence predates essence' and, given existentialism's influence on nursing theory and on patient-centred approaches to care, it may be worth considering it in a little more detail.

The existential position is basically this – that a person 'comes in to existence' and that a person's 'essence' or 'personhood' only emerges later. The 'essence' is whatever that person makes it. He or she is the 'author of his or her essence'. For Sartre, a person is both free and responsible. He or she is free to become whatever he or she makes of him or herself. Because of that freedom, the person is also responsible for what he or she becomes. We cannot be free and *not* responsible.

While people are free to make decisions, they must also consider the *responsibility* that goes with such behaviour. Like it or not, other people will be affected by our actions: our spouses, children, friends, work colleagues, and so on.

All this leads us back to the process of caring. We continue to care because we continue to endorse care as 'right action'. We may feel different tomorrow, so our beliefs and judgments may change as we evolve as people, but for now we believe that caring is important. Furthermore, we hope that other people's actions – in as far as they affect us – will also involve caring. We hope that others will care for us, although we cannot guarantee that they will.

One of the most liberating – if daunting – features of existentialism is its *dynamic* quality. People, as defined by existentialists, are always in a state of flux: they are always engaged in the process of *becoming*. The human project is never complete. In this sense, we can never define, once and for all, what we *should* or *must* do. All we can do is to continue to review and reaffirm our beliefs – almost on a day-to-day basis. Caring, in this sense, becomes something of an act of faith that influences every aspect of our lives.

❏ The spiritual aspect

The whole issue of to what 'spirituality' might be referring is a complex one. While the word itself contains another word, 'spirit', the term has been used more broadly than one to connote simply a belief in the inherent *spirit* of a person. It is, however, most frequently linked to religion and to religious beliefs.

We mentioned earlier that a common theme in many religions is the need for members of the faith to *care* for one another. In all of the major world religions, this idea of caring for each other is paramount. Indeed, it would be difficult to imagine a religion that suggested otherwise. To *care*, therefore, has become an essential 'regulation' of religious faiths.

It follows, therefore, that the 'religious' nurse is also one who cares, not because he or she is a *nurse* but rather because he or she is a member of that religion or faith. Most religions have a 'code of conduct' – usually written into holy books – that *prescribes* care for others. To care, in this case, is to follow the teachings of that particular religion by reference to its code of conduct. In this sense, the religious view of caring is very much akin to the *moral* view of caring.

However, not every nurse has a commitment to some form of religion that may generate a desire to care for others, and this is where the notion of spirituality comes in. It is possible for people to believe that caring for others is the right thing to do even if they do not believe in religion.

It is quite possible to argue that many people care simply because they choose to do so. Why? Possibly because caring is itself *enjoyable.* In all the rather heavy debate about motives, attitudes, spiritual and non-spiritual issues, it is sometimes possible to lose sight of the sheer pleasure that caring for others can give.

However it is viewed, it would seem that caring is an almost universal phenomenon, one linked to the very process of becoming and being a person. If that is the case, caring remains at the centre of the process of nursing for, whatever it is *not,* nursing *is* intimately bound up with all aspects of the person.

■ Applications

These theories may be important as we develop new curriculum ideas and documents in the future. They may elicit a change in the content and process of nurse education so that *caring* and *communicating* are emphasised more forcefully.

■ Summary

This chapter has explored the nature of caring – particularly from the point of view of Campbell's analysis. It has also examined a variety of other definitions of it and noted the tension between caring in theory and caring in practice. The chapter closed with a brief debate about the relationship between caring and nursing and the question was posed, 'Why should nurses care?' In the next chapter, we explore further the nature of caring by broadening the discussion to include the notions of altruism and helping behaviour.

Whatever our views on caring, it is essential that we are at all times clear about the *language* we use to describe it. Radsma (1994) offers this timely and appropriate observation about the nature of the caring literature:

> The fact that caring is a human need is indisputable. That caring is at the root of nursing history is also unquestionable. That caring is the essence of nursing must yet be determined. Nursing cannot continue to use the linguistics of care without an explicit and implicit understanding of what professional caring entails.

■ Further reading

Chalmers, K.J. and Luker, K.A. 1992 The development of the health visitor–client relationship. *Scandinavian Journal of Caring Sciences,* **5**:33–41.

Elstad, J.I. 1994 Women's priorities regarding physician behavior and their preference for a female physician. *Women and Health,* **2**(4):1–19.

Fink, S.V. 1995 The influence of family resources and family demands on the strains and well-being of caregiving families. *Nursing Research,* **44**(3):139–46.

Jivanjee, P. 1994 Enhancing the well-being of family caregivers to patients with Alzheimer's disease. *Journal of Gerontological Social Work,* **23**(1/2):31–48.

Kurtz, M.E., Kurtz, J.C., Given, C.W. and Given, B. 1995 Relationship of caregiver reactions and depression to cancer patients' symptoms, functional states and depression – a longitudinal view. *Social Science and Medicine,* **40**(6):837–46.

Lewis, L. 1995 Caring for the carers. *Modern Midwife,* **5**(2):7–10.

McDrury, J. 1994 Client satisfaction in the community setting: a review of literature. *New Zealand Practice Nurse,* September, 92–3.

Neufeld, A. and Harrison, M.J. 1995 Reciprocity and social support in caregivers' relationships: variations and consequences. *Qualitative Health Research,* **5**(3): 348–65.

Norrby, E. and Bellner, A. 1995 The helping encounter: occupational therapists' perception of therapeutic relationships. *Scandinavian Journal of Caring Sciences,* **9**(1):41–6.

Picot, S.J. 1995 Rewards, costs, and coping of African American caregivers. *Nursing Research,* **44**(3):147–52.

Small, E. 1995 Valuing the unseen emotional labour of nursing. *Nursing Times,* **91**(26):40–1.

Sofaer, B. 1994 Achieving a better life on the planet. Are we our 'brothers' keepers'? *Nursing Ethics: An International Journal for Health Care Professionals,* **1**(3):173–7.

Taylor, R., Ford, G. and Dunbar, M. 1995 The effects of caring on health: a community based longitudinal study. *Social Science and Medicine,* **40**(10):1407–15.

Tishelman, C. 1994 Cancer patient's hopes and expectations of nursing practice in Stockholm – patients' descriptions and nursing discourse. *Scandinavian Journal of Caring Science,* **8**(4):213–22.

Toseland, R.W., Blanchard, C.G. and McCallion, P. 1995 A problem solving intervention for caregivers of cancer patients. *Social Science and Medicine,* **40**(4):517–28.

Chapter Two

Psychological care in nursing

As we noted in the previous chapter, the word 'caring' is a term familiar to all the helping professions. The literature frequently refers to caring relationships and stresses the importance of caring in the helping role. Yet relatively few studies have been carried out to explore what caring means for the nurses who do it on a day-to-day basis. If nursing is *the* caring profession, a great deal of research needs to be carried out into what caring is and how it affects the professional nursing carer. One approach to exploring caring is through an examination of the *psychological* care of the patient.

It will be useful to explore some of the wider theoretical frameworks and to discuss briefly some of the key concepts which may be applied to the process of caring in nursing practice. The general field of research is the field of altruism and helping behaviour. Caring is another process which fits in nicely here. This area has been one of the central areas of research in social psychology over the past 30 years. A number of important theories and concepts have been generated from research in the field which need to be mentioned, and these have been summarised below.

■ Attribution theory

Attribution theory deals with the ways in which people attribute causes to their own behaviour and the behaviour of other people in a social context. People generally wish to know *why* they acted in a certain way under certain conditions. The theoretical foundations for this are outlined in the work of Heider (1958), later influential developments in the theory being found in the work of Jones and Davis (1965) and Kelley (1972).

Jones and Davis (1965), while emphasising internal motivation, were concerned with the way in which we infer lasting characteristics of people from their behaviour. They suggested that we do so by focusing attention on the specific types of action which are likely to be most informative. The process, however, is more prominent when the actions of the individual occur under certain conditions:

- the action is freely chosen
- it produces outcomes which may not be produced by any other deed, and
- it is perceived as low in terms of social desirability.

Kelley (1972), on the other hand, focused on the cause of an event or course of action. In Kelley's theory, we look for explanations of people's behaviour by attending to three distinct dimensions. In the first place, we refer to the notion of *consensus* – that is, the extent to which others in the same situation act in the same manner. The second process we refer to is that of *consistency*, which is the extent to which a person reacts in a constant manner to a similar set of circumstances. Finally, the notion of *distinctiveness* is the degree to which a person behaves in a similar manner to different sets of circumstances.

As the conditions of these three dimensions change, so too does the way in which people make attributions about behaviour. For example, Kelley suggested that under conditions of low consensus, high consistency and low distinctiveness, internal causes of behaviour will be attributed. An example here may be the way in which a particular nurse may react to patients with sexually transmitted diseases. The conditions here might be as follows: low consensus (other nurses do not react negatively to the patient and his family); high consistency (the nurse responds negatively to all patients with sexually transmitted diseases in a similar and negative way); and low distinctiveness (the nurse reacts negatively to patients with different problems). Under these conditions, we would expect the nurse to suggest that the patient is responsible for his or her own ill health.

On the other hand, external causes will be attributed where there is a profile of high consistency, high consensus and high distinctiveness. The approach has also been used, in the form of Bem's theory of self-perception (Bem, 1972), to describe the ways in which we attribute causes of our own behaviour. In this way, we make inferences about our own behaviour just as we do about the behaviour of other people.

The attribution theory approach has been successfully applied to a range of social problems, including attempts to reduce interpersonal conflict (Baron, 1985); promoting an understanding of people's reactions to the victims of serious crimes such as rape (Kanekar *et al.*, 1985); in the field of marital difficulties (Holtzworth-Munroe and Jacobson, 1985); and with learning difficulties (Wilson and Linville, 1982). In addition, this approach has been recognised as an important strategy in psychological research in the study of ordinary explanations of social behaviour (Harris and Harvey, 1981; Lalljee, 1981). The importance and relevance of the *context* in which attributions are made has also been emphasised (Harris and Harvey, 1981).

In studies of helping behaviour, attribution theory has been used to explore the mediating role that *affect* has on helping (Weiner, 1980). Weiner found that when an individual perceived another person to be in need of help, he or she usually attributed the cause of the distress to internal or external factors. Where an internal or controllable cause was attributed by the observer, feelings of anger or disgust were elicited and help was refused. On the other hand, if external or uncontrollable causes of the distress were attributed, feelings of sympathy and concern were elicited in the observer and help was more likely to be given. A number of other empirical studies offer support for this general theory (Barnes *et al.*, 1979; Meyer and Mulherin, 1980).

■ The social learning approach

In this approach, helping may be defined as a process that is learned from other people through the mechanisms of reinforcement, observation and role modelling. Helping behaviour may be conditioned by reinforcement, whereas unsociable behaviour may be punished (Rushton, 1980).

The social learning approach has been found to be especially useful in studies which explore how children learn to be helpful and caring. Fisher (1963), for example, found that reinforcement could be used to increase sharing behaviour in 4-year-old children. Other studies have also reported that helping and altruistic behaviour can be facilitated through good role models (Eisenberg-Berg and Geisheker, 1979).

It is notable that, in a professional context, established team members play an important role in the training and education of learners and untrained staff. They are important role model figures. The ward sister is perhaps the best example of this. Think for a moment of how often you have tried to emulate those ward sisters or charge nurses you perceived to be effective and caring individuals.

■ The cognitive development approach

This approach also emphasises the learning process in helping behaviour, but instead of stressing the external or environmental aspects of learning, it highlights the cognitive changes that occur as the individual develops. These changes may be seen as a series of stages, the later ones reflecting more complex and advanced forms of thinking, reasoning, decision-making and problem-solving, and being essential cognitive activities influencing the individual's willingness to help others.

In addition, as the individual develops, so too does the ability for moral reasoning and the capacity for helping behaviour, which is believed to reflect the individual's overall cognitive development (Krebs, 1978). Some studies have reported higher rates of helping with higher levels of moral reasoning (Harris *et al.*, 1976).

■ Other approaches to helping

In contrast to some of the broader theoretical frameworks outlined above, other approaches have been developed which emphasise some of the relatively distinct variables that may be used to predict helping in a variety of settings. Two major trends can be identified: (1) studies which attempt to identify stable personal characteristics or traits in the helper, and (2) other studies which address the distinctive properties of the particular setting in which help is given. The personal characteristics are usually assessed through the use of attitude scales, such as those that attempt to measure empathy.

Some of the personal dimensions which have been found consistently to relate to helping behaviour are personal norms (a sense of moral obligation to help) (Schwartz, 1977) and empathy (Coke *et al.*, 1978). In contrast, the situational correlates of helping include how serious the helper perceives the situation to be, what possible cost will be incurred by the helper and the perceived competence of other available helpers. These situational factors have been found to determine whether or not help is given (Smithson *et al.*, 1983). The emphasis in this approach is on employing specific scales or other measures and establishing statistical correlations between these variables and the help given.

■ Some problems of research on altruism and helping

Although a large number of studies in this field have been already been completed, some writers have been very critical of the approach used in the research. There has been a dominance of positivist methodology influencing most of the models described above, and it has been of limited use in applied fields such as teaching, medicine, nursing and other helping professions. Pearce *et al.* (1983) summarised this important trend as follows:

> The dominant tradition in social psychological research has been an experimental, laboratory-based mode of inquiry. Researchers using this approach attempt to understand important social behaviour through the control and

manipulation of factors which influence simulated forms of the target behaviours. This research reflects a positivist philosophy of science and a limited deterministic view of human action.

Consequently, much of the research completed to date has been criticised on the grounds of having low external validity in the real world, having a limited perception of human action, lacking a cumulative body of research and being politically and socially conservative (Pearce *et al.*, 1983). In addition, in those studies where realistic field settings have been used, there has been a tendency to use:

> small inconsequential helping acts to represent large scale phenomena such as caring and empathy. (Pearce *et al.*, 1983)

In the next section, we begin to explore some of the research on caring, which has moved out from the laboratory and into the world of work. Very little research has been completed which focuses on helping and caring behaviour in a *professional* context, but this is the sort of research that is needed if new theoretical perspectives are to be developed which have implications for educators, researchers and practising nurses.

■ Research into caring

A number of nurse researchers have attempted to investigate the process of caring, but most of these have been completed in an American context. Few British studies can be found in the literature. Some of American research studies are reviewed briefly below, but the findings must be considered carefully because of the wide discrepancies between health care philosophies, facilities and practices in these different cultures. Kyle (1995) offers a more detailed literature review of the concept of caring, and the sample offered here is only a small review of some of the work that has been done in this field.

Using a qualitative anthropological design, Leininger (1977) studied the process of caring across a range of cultures over a 15-year period. Data from almost 30 different cultures were collected. Variations in the belief and value systems of the informants, as well as variations in the practice of caring across these cultural settings, were uncovered.

Leininger classified a total of 17 constructs (or 'ways of perceiving') related to caring: comfort, support, compassion, empathy, direct helping behaviours, coping, specific stress alleviation, touching, nurturance, succorance, surveillance, protection, restoration, stimulation, health maintenance, health instruction and health consultation. As the research evolved, these were subsequently developed into a 28-construct taxonomy of caring.

Unfortunately, many details of the research methods that she used were not reported, and this makes it very difficult to check how reliable and valid her findings were. However, the fact that different constructs were found to be more significant across cultures is particularly important and should caution researchers against the dangers of trying to produce a universal description of caring.

■ The patient's view of caring

Another approach to the issue of what caring is, is to ask those people who have recently received care what it was like. This was the strategy used by Henry (1975). She employed open-ended interviews with 50 people who had recently received nursing care, and later devised three major categories for classifying caring nurse behaviours:

1. what the nurse does
2. how the nurse does, and
3. how much the nurse does.

Remarkably, very similar findings were reported in a study by Brown (1982). Again, patients were interviewed and asked to describe a specific time or an incident in which they felt cared for by a nurse. The responses were analysed into different categories or content areas using content analysis, and two themes were revealed:

1. what the nurse does, and
2. what the nurse is like.

Brown also asked the respondents in the study to fill in a Likert rating scale in order to assess the importance of the 'task' and 'affective' components of the care that they had received. These were then analysed using a statistical procedure, and the results revealed that patients perceived both these dimensions to be equally important.

Note how the different approaches in the research have resulted in quite diverse descriptions of what caring means to the people involved in the studies. This highlights the need to include a range of perspectives if we are to arrive at a description of caring which can be put to work in a number of dimensions of nursing, for example evaluating standards of care, teaching and training, consumer studies, and so on.

In another study, patient perceptions of caring behaviours have also been explored in oncology nursing using the Q-sort technique (Larson, 1984), which is a means of exploring people's perceptions through the use of statements on cards. Each person is given a pack of such cards and asked to sort the statements into 'sets' of (usually) seven assortments of cards, ranging from one that represents one extreme of a continuum to a pile that represents the other extreme. The researcher using the technique gives the respondent labels for the two ends of the continuum. Thus, in a study of aspects of self, Nyatanga (1989) used the extremes of 'most like me' and 'least like me' to explore respondents' perceptions of self.

In the Q-sort study described by Larson, patients reported that the most important caring behaviours which they observed in nurses were:

- accessibility (checking patients frequently, responding quickly to call alarms, and so on), and
- monitoring and follow-through (knowing when to call a doctor, how to give an injection and how to manage equipment).

Larson (1984) found that the patients' view of caring was quite different from that of the nurses working in the oncology area, who ranked 'listening' and 'comfort' as its most important components. The study provides further evidence of the need for more research into human concepts such as comfort, caring and listening. In addition, Larson cautions that:

Listening and talking, psychosocial skills highly valued by nurses, appear to become important to these patients only after their basic 'getting better' needs are met. (Larson, 1984, p. 50)

The evidence seems to suggest that the most valuable insights into the caring process must include a patient perspective and a nursing perspective. Relatives, too, are another important group who will be able to provide meaningful insights into the caring process (Nolan and Grant, 1989).

There is a need for nurse researchers and nurse educators to take into account the 'larger canvas'. We cannot concentrate only on teaching and learning specific practical and interpersonal skills. We must also consider the views of patients, their relatives and other health care workers, and also those less tangible aspects of nursing: comfort, caring, empathy and understanding. By taking account of these factors, nursing researchers and educators can continue to inform and develop nursing practice.

■ The nurse's view of caring

In contrast to the patient perspective, Ford (1981) asked a sample of nearly 200 nurses to define caring in their own words and to describe their own caring behaviours. A questionnaire was used to collect the data. Data analysis revealed two major categories which reflected: (1) a genuine concern for the well-being of another, and (2) giving of oneself.

Some examples of the caring behaviours provided by the nurses in the study were listening, helping and showing respect, and supporting the actions of others. The nurses' view failed to emphasise those 'task' dimensions stressed in other studies involving patient perceptions, such as the one reported by Brown (1982) mentioned above.

Forrest (1989) provided a phenomenological analysis of nurses' experiences of caring for patients. The phenomenological approach is characterised by its emphasis on the lived experience. It attempts to understand the phenomenon (in this case caring for another person) from the perspective of those individuals being studied. The accent is on depth rather than on the quantity of data collected, and very strict procedures of analysis must be adhered to. In this study, only 17 informants were engaged. Two major categories of response were identified: (1) what is caring?, and (2) what affects caring?

The first category, 'what is caring?', was broken down further into two sub-categories – involvement and interacting. The second category, 'what affects caring?', was broken down into a further five themes. These included: oneself, the patient, frustrations, coping and comfort, and support. Again, note how the different approach to the problem influences the type of data that emerges from the research. With very qualitative and in-depth strategies, very detailed descriptions have emerged which convey some of the complex factors that influence caring in nursing.

■ Other views of caring in nursing

As an alternative to asking patients or nurses for their views about caring, Ray (1981b) used the method of participant observation, which entailed observing people at work and exploring their roles, clinical units and documents. Participant observation is a research technique in which the researcher takes herself into the research field and not only observes what is going on, but also takes part in the day-to-day action that occurs. Ray observed caring in the clinical setting and identified 1362 caring responses. When these were analysed, a conceptual classification system of caring was produced which had four important categories. These were:

1. psychological (cognitive and affective)
2. practical (technical and social organisation)
3. interactional (social and physical), and
4. philosophical (spiritual, ethical and cultural).

The practical aspects of caring were again very evident in this study.

In summary, few research studies of the meaning of caring have been carried out in the field of nursing. While some of these have examined patients' views, others have attempted to explore the nurses' perspective. Differences in the ways in which nurses and patients perceive caring appear to be emerging, but these require further exploration and description.

■ Psychological care of patients

In 1953 the Nuffield Provincial Hospitals Trust defined 'nursing care' as 'activities required to provide the physical, medical, and emotional needs of the patient'. The term 'psychological' may be substituted for 'emotional' here. It could be argued that many of the developments that have occurred in the organisation of nursing work, such as 'team nursing', 'patient allocation' or 'primary nursing', have been implemented to improve nurses' and patients' levels of satisfaction with interpersonal communication and emotional/psychological care.

Some writers in this area have attempted to draw together many aspects of nursing care that could be construed as psychological care, so we will briefly examine a few of these. The first of these was produced recently by John Hall (1990), a clinical psychologist who proposed that the term 'care' has four major components:

1. a set of beliefs or philosophies that may be unarticulated which guide what people do
2. a set of objectives developed from a philosophy and an analysis of people's needs
3. a set of acts which emphasise what happens in a caring encounter, and
4. the emotions and feelings that accompany care.

> Care is a mutual process in that the cared-for and the carer either actively or passively engage in the caring encounter or interaction, which may be non-verbal, verbal or behavioural. (Hall, 1990, p. 133)

Hall's analysis of 'caring' is very general and can only be considered as an outline to stimulate discussion in this area.

The next approach was also developed by a psychologist with a commitment to training nurses (Nichols, 1985). He suggested that psychological care involved:

- monitoring the psychological state
- representing the patient's psychological needs (acting on behalf of the patient)
- emotional care
- informational care

- basic counselling skills, and
- co-support and case discussion.

Nichol's approach has a lot more substance than does Hall's. Each of his components is one of 'psychological care', and he has also identified the need to set these out within the organisational structure in which health care is given. This is a very important point for, as we will see a little later on, the organisational structures and culture appear to play an important role in determining the sort of psychological care that patients receive.

❏ Affective and instrumental components of care

Ben-Sira (1976, 1980, 1983), in a series of Israeli studies into patients' satisfaction with care, highlighted the importance of the doctors' and nurses' affective behaviour because it influenced patients' perceptions of the hospital and the competence of the staff, and ultimately patients' recovery from illness.

Affective behaviour in this instance means giving 'time' to the patient, showing an 'interest' in the patient's personal problems and being 'devoted' to the management of these. However, there may be a discrepancy between *patients'* and *nurses'* views of caring, which probably vary both across cultures and across nursing specialities (mental health, oncology, surgery, for example). Clifford (1995), in an analysis of caring from the practice perspective, makes the following point:

> It may be that the tendency for patients to perceive the instrumental role of caring as most important is simply a reaction to the realities of health-care provision, whilst nurses identifying the importance of the affective role are seeking an ideal that is not possible in organised health care today.

The relative importance of the instrumental and expressive components of care has not been satisfactorily demonstrated. One view is that both these components are very important to patients and their families.

❏ Patient satisfaction

Research has shown that satisfied patients are more likely to comply with medical regimes (DiMatteo and DiNicola, 1982) and that nurses have an important role to play in passing on and reinforcing instructions, and in becoming agents of health promotion.

It is important to understand the patients' points of view (Posner, 1994) in order to deal effectively with their individual concerns. Johnson and Jones (1979) construed the process of 'recovery' as being restored psychological well-being after medical treatment:

> The healing of illness requires more than healing parts of the body; it requires intensive efforts to communicate with patients. (Reiser, 1978, p. 23)

Patients who are satisfied with professional care are more likely to use services in the future (Roghmann *et al.*, 1979), so good psychological care may make a significant difference to consumers. Another focus in the literature is on the concept of learned helplessness in hospitals. Studies of patients' experiences during hospitalisation support the view that learned helplessness describes very well the psychological state that many patients assume. The care of these patients has an essentially psychological perspective, of which nurses need to be aware.

■ Learned helplessness in hospitals

Taylor (1979) has argued that when patients become 'patients', they 'present' themselves in three distinct modes. These modes of identity may be influenced by the person's personality, previous experience of hospitalisation, length of their stay in hospital and expectations of hospital and the service. People as patients may present themselves as: (1) non-discriminant, (2) compliant, or (3) difficult and demanding.

❏ The non-discriminant patient

This reaction is probably a response to the hospital systems that 'depersonalise' people/patients through bureaucratic routines and impersonal treatment from the nursing and medical staff. Patients may try unsuccessfully to gain control over the situation by getting information from any of a large number of staff (30 or so) with whom they come into contact each day. Patients become increasingly anxious about their situation.

❏ The compliant patient

The compliant patient is, according to Taylor, denying the awful circumstances of hospital, presenting a self that appears to be undisturbed by hospital, illness and suffering, and ready to help the staff in whatever way possible. The compliant patient feels powerless and helpless. He or she may harbour feelings of anxiety and hostility.

❏ The difficult and demanding patient

The difficult and demanding patient expresses anger about the illness, its implications or the manner in which he or she has been treated in hospital. The anger may be expressed as 'petty mutiny', such as defiance of some of the hospital rules, or it may ultimately lead to dangerous behaviours such as failing to take important medications. Taylor (1979) commented that hospitals are 'unpleasant places to be' (p. 156), and the loss of control over important life events leads to 'depersonalisation' (Goffman, 1961). Raps *et al.* (1982) tested 48 inpatients hospitalised for 1, 3 and 9 weeks and 24 outpatients on cognitive tasks and found that poor performance and symptoms of depression increased with length of stay in hospital, even as the patient's condition improved.

It is interesting to ask *why* patients present themselves in these ways. Raps *et al.* (1982) claim that, while administering a 'cure' to patients, the institutional nature of hospital life may cause learned helplessness that can impede cure and recovery. In addition, helplessness may elicit more caring responses from nurses (Morrison, 1992). We now move on to another area that raises cause for concern: that to do with the relationship between physical and psychological care.

■ Physical care and psychological care

Hall (1966) argued that the need to provide physical care to the patient allowed the nurse to be an effective teacher and nurturer. There appears to be a move away from the importance of physical care, as can be seen in the work of several nursing theorists, for example Jean Watson (Dunlop, 1986).

Stannard (1973) carried out a participant observation study of the nursing care given to people in an old folks home. He found that the 'nurses' had little direct contact with patients; they did not do any of the 'dirty work'. Instead they administered, organised, co-ordinated and directed the activities of the aides who took care of the patients' needs. This general approach meant that a 'custodial' ideology dominated the care of the old folk, who were often 'abused' by the aides. Abuse here means pulling a patient's hair, slapping, hitting, pinching or shaking the patient violently.

■ Basic care is carried out by the least well-prepared staff

There is also a need to look carefully at who does what in practice. Who provides the basic/physical care in general hospital settings? Knight and

Field's (1981) study of dying cancer patients on an acute surgical ward vividly portrayed how the most junior and inexperienced members of the staff had the most contact with patients through providing their basic care.

As a result these members of staff had to 'deal with' the dying patient as best they could. The authors claimed that the system of organising medical and nursing care was at fault. This was also the finding of New *et al.* (1959) – that aides did most of the basic care. This pattern of work was also found to exist in small study of German nurses (Morrison and Bauer, 1993).

These findings pose particular problems for those nurses offering direct care. Other studies have observed the stresses imposed on younger staff who have the greatest contact with patients (Jacobson and McGrath, 1983; Livingston and Livingston, 1984). The least well-prepared and least experienced staff have to cope with a very demanding role – they may not cope well with patients; they may, personally, find it all too much.

■ Information-giving in patient care

The next section deals with information-giving as a component of psychological care – informational care of the patient and his or her family. The positive effect of information and encouragement has been recognised for over 30 years (see for example Egbert *et al.*, 1964; Skipper and Leonard, 1968).

Research has clearly demonstrated that giving patients information about their management and care is a very effective strategy in terms of both patient satisfaction with care and cost-effectiveness. However, it is not essential that nurses provide information – other members of the team can also do a good job here.

Moreover, a number of studies of trained and untrained nurses have shown that these staff perceive themselves as being 'good' providers of information. However, it must noted that most complaints about care have to do with poor communication between staff, patients and relatives, or between the staff themselves. The Audit Commission (1993) high-lighted lack of information and problems in communication with health professionals as being at the top of the list of patient concerns.

■ The importance of the physical environment

The physical environment is also an important component of patient satisfaction and a contributing factor in helping to provide good psychological care; this has been studied in over 23 hospitals by Kenny and Canter (1979). The physical environment is likely also to influence patient psychological well-being while in hospital. The hospital environment is an alien one and generates much anxiety in patients and their families (Leigh and Reiser, 1980). Nurses should not underestimate the importance that patients place on the environment and hotel facilities.

■ Activity analysis of nursing work

Wallis (1987) and others completed a programme of research on job satisfaction among nurses in South Wales in the 1980s. They used a variety of methods, including direct observation of behaviour, activity sampling, participant observation, the introduction of differently organised tasks for staff, interviews, records and questionnaires, scales of job satisfaction and attitudes. Wallis (1987) reported that all levels of nursing staff reported a high level of job satisfaction, but a number of important sources of dissatisfaction and frustration were also noted.

It appeared that nurses were highly motivated by patients' *total dependence* on them and enjoyed their 'caring' role. Yet the nurses claimed that they were prevented from spending time with patients. Their efforts to provide good care were undermined by inadequate resources and administrative incompetence, being subject to 'distant' medical control.

The nurses in these studies of psychogeriatric patients focused their efforts on 'physical care', which meant that patients became very dependent (Tables 2.1 and 2.2). A number of aspects of the nurses' role were seen as 'good': keeping busy, doing things for other people, social relationships with other staff, having good supervisors, doing interesting work, having variety and the occasional sense of achievement that the work presented. A number of aspects were seen as 'bad': staff shortages, the lack of time to provide optimal care for patients, poor communication with management and non-involvement in decisions on how to spend money within the hospital.

Table 2.1   Activity sampling analysis of nursing staff activities. Percentages of time on ward at these activities (Adapted from Wallis, 1987 and Cope, 1981)

	Ward A (Male)	Ward B (Female)
Physical care	59.0	52.0
Psychological care	6.4	14.1
Administrative breaks	28.8	30.6
Miscellaneous	5.7	3.4

Psychological care involved talking to patients, playing games such as cards, doing jigsaw puzzles, and so on. Physical care included dressing, washing, toileting, bed-making and preparing patients for treatment. Administration meant time spent away from the ward, communication with other staff, tea breaks and so on. In terms of patient activities, 'non-purposeful activity' referred to being awake but doing nothing, being asleep or sitting with eyes closed, wandering around the ward, and so on. Purposeful activity included watching TV and smoking! These findings may say a lot about the *quality of psychological* care offered to these patients.

Table 2.2   Activity sampling analysis of patients (psychogeriatric). Percentages of time spent in ward at these activities (Adapted from Wallis, 1987 and Cope, 1981)

	Ward A (Male)	Ward B (Female)
Non-purposeful activity	71.3	76.2
Purposeful activity	6.9	1.7
Physical maintenance	14.0	8.8
Toilet behaviour	2.9	0.8
Social interaction	4.6	12.4

A number of innovations to improve the situation were introduced. One of these was the 'total patient care' system, giving each nurse greater responsibility for a smaller group of patients and for completing all important aspects of that patient's care. This innovation did not lead to the predicted changes in satisfaction, and the system was dropped because 'it was not in the patients' best interests' (Wallis, 1987, p. 120).

It was suggested that the lack of agreed social and psychological objectives for this type of care meant that the nurses 'felt under no pressure to behave in ways which would show as much regard and priority for remedial and therapeutic psychological care, as for physical and custodial care' (p. 121).

■ Does an increase in the number of staff make a difference?

Moores and Grant (1977) studied the pattern of interaction in two hospitals (one well, the other poorly resourced) for mentally handicapped patients and found that patients who exhibited the greatest maladaptive behaviour received more attention, although the type of attention received (essentially containment) was not likely to lead to improvements in behaviour.

A similar finding has been documented in Altschul's analysis of psychiatric nursing in 1972 – the most difficult patients received the most interaction from staff, and some patients did not interact with staff at all.

Perhaps these nurses have developed a 'problem-solving' approach to their work and more visible problems are prioritised. In a very early study of nurse staffing levels on medical and surgical wards, New et al. (1959) found that when more staff nurses were introduced onto the wards, the nurses did not on the whole spend more time interacting with patients: they chose to do other things.

■ Does the organisational culture influence staff?

Studies of care must be contextualised (institution or community, working as a member of a group, working as an individual). Peterson (1988) attempted to address the problem of the poor psychological care given to patients by examining the norms and values upon which nursing work is based in three groups of nurses on different units. A qualitative approach using grounded theory was employed.

1. She found that each of three groups was influenced by group norms and values. Nurses who were atypical were penalised for this deviance in various subtle ways, for example being given a heavier workload.
2. In addition, the group leader was very influential in setting the group norms and values – some set the tone of the ward by focusing on getting through the work 'on time', and this generated a tense, rushed atmosphere.
3. On all three units, typical care was centred on physical care of the patient, technical procedures and giving medication.
4. This study emphasises the importance of the organisational culture as a major determinant of nursing work.

■ Is it a training problem?

Although there has been a huge emphasis on interpersonal skills training and communication in health care, we are not convinced that a lack of training is solely responsible for this problem. It may be possible to train people in important interpersonal skills such as listening and to make them more aware of their own prejudices and values. However, the results of this training may be short lived. When these individuals are placed in the 'organisation' as 'workers', they quickly learn to acquire the dominant norms and values prevailing within that institution – thus undermining any earlier training. Moreover, the type of training that students are exposed to may not be ideally suited to the demands of the professional worker. Studies of 'informal' helpers suggest that they can do a very successful job in helping people to deal with psychological problems –

social interaction skills, ordinariness in human interaction, may be just as important as 'interpersonal skills'.

Cowen (1982) summarised findings from a series of studies of informal helpers: hairdressers, divorce lawyers, industrial supervisors and bartenders. Many of the problems areas raised with these groups were similar to those that clients raised with mental health professionals: difficulties with children, physical health, marital problems, depression, anxiety, financial and emotional problems, and so on. Most of the respondents felt good about providing interpersonal help and believed that they did a good job.

These informal helpers adopted a number of strategies to help their clients: they offered support and sympathy, they tried to be light-hearted, they just listened, they presented alternatives, they shared personal experiences, they tried not to get involved, they gave advice, they tried to change the topic, and so on. They offered a spontaneous response highlighting their humanity and ordinariness – nurse training works in a different way.

■ The need for change and reactions to change

If nurses are serious about the importance of psychological care for patients and their families, they must think carefully about how to operationalise that objective in the future. Clearly, while many of the developments that have taken place over the last few decades have benefited patients, the whole business of psychological care is rather unclear, and the standards of psychological care are variable and inconsistent. There is a need to look for the hidden values of managers and practitioners that influence the way in which nurses work. Almost 40 years ago, Sofer made the following observation:

> If behavioural modes persist through time, this is usually because they continue to fulfil functions for the organisation or individuals concerned, sometimes even unknown to the latter. Administrative edicts can change formal organisation, but cannot work while interaction is still geared to prior rules and underpinned by established values. (Sofer, 1955, pp. 300–1)

■ Achieving change in nursing practice

Change must be of an evolutionary rather than revolutionary nature. Perhaps we are trying to change too rapidly. That is why many of the innovations that have sprung up overnight in nursing do not work. They have not been thought through properly, they are not guided by research, and little or no account is taken of how to promote effective change in people's working lives. Henneman (1984) suggested that:

To change a system it is essential to understand something of its nature. Success is unlikely if you proceed on the basis of what *should be* the case... [and] sustained change is more reliably achieved by a process of guided evolution than by hero-innovator catalysed revolution. (pp. 14, 16)

■ Who should provide psychological care?

There is another important issue that the profession needs to address: 'who' should provide psychological care for patients and their families? Some years ago Wilson (1950) said that:

Insofar as the increased interest in the patient as a person represents a continuing trend... it is clear that hospitals will in future need to consider some increase in the size of that part of the staff which is primarily concerned with the patient as a person. In theory, staff for such purposes might be either trained nurses or nursing auxiliaries... on grounds of availability and for other reasons, nursing auxiliaries are more likely to be used in such a development immediately and in the future. (Wilson, 1950, p. 91)

From the account provided here, this view is as relevant today as it was over 40 years ago. Perhaps the profession has lost its way in the drive towards 'professionalisation'. Perhaps practising nurses are not really interested in the 'basic' care that provides opportunities for good psychological care.

The view that the psychological care of the patient may be undertaken by aides continues to be relevant in today's climate. It would seem that a move towards training aides or helpers in this area would prove cost-effective and probably lead to significant improvements in consumer satisfaction.

Care and attention must urgently be afforded to this issue. We really need to clarify the trained nurse's role in this area if we are to lift the cloud of confusion that surrounds psychological care of the patient. Only then we will be truly able to offer the type of psychological care that patients need.

■ Personal construct theory and nurses' perceptions of caring

In the study described here we set out to explore nurses' perceptions of the meaning of caring in nursing practice. Kellys' Personal Construct Theory (PCT), (Kelly, 1955; Bannister and Fransella, 1986) and the repertory grid technique were used. The repertory grid technique has the advantage of being flexible enough to combine both qualitative and quantitative data, but in this chapter its qualitative aspects will be emphasised. It may be helpful to explore briefly some of the key aspects of the repertory grid approach. Rawlinson (1995) offers a useful review of the applications of this approach to other nursing settings, and Taylor (1990) describes various alternative ways of analysing repertory grid data.

❏ Repertory grid technique

Repertory grid techniques were developed out of George Kelly's (1955, 1963, 1969; Adams-Webber, 1979) theory of personal constructs. Kelly argued that each individual views the world through what Bannister, Fransella and Kelly call a particular 'pair of psychological goggles' (Bannister and Fransella, 1986). People's views of the world are coloured by their personal experiences, background, culture, education, belief and value systems, and so on. There is no 'objective' view of the world that can be apprehended by any particular individual. Each person views the world idiosyncratically.

The theory that Kelly offers is a fairly elaborate one that is described in detail elsewhere (Bannister and Mair 1968; Fransella and Bannister, 1977). The interested reader will find these texts particularly helpful. The repertory grid technique, devised by Kelly, offers one approach to identifying how individuals perceive people and the world around them. It offers the researcher a method of systematically exploring and recording an individual's world. The method has been used for research in a wide number of areas from counselling and psychotherapy (Epting, 1984) to education (Beail, 1985), to industrial and commercial settings (Stewart and Stewart, 1981). Here, our aim is to consider some of the practical implications of Kelly's repertory grid technique as it relates to nursing research.

Applications of the grid technique

Although personal construct theory and the repertory grid technique were developed from the clinical field, they have been relatively infrequently applied in nursing research. There are a few notable studies, however, which should be mentioned.

Wilkinson (1982) used the grid technique to examine attitude changes in general nursing students towards psychiatric patients. While Davis (1983) explored the formal and informal aspects of nurse training using the repertory grid method, Heyman *et al.* (1983) investigated the socialisation process of nursing trainees in British hospitals, and Costigan *et al.* (1987) used the grid technique to explore nurses' perceptions of attempted suicide. Most recently, Pollock (1987) employed the technique to study the role of the community psychiatric nurse.

❏ Sample of nurses

A sample of 25 informants was selected to participate in the study. The ward sister/charge nurse group was pinpointed as being the most relevant starting point. This specialist group has been found to be influential in determining educational and training opportunities at ward level (Orton, 1981; Marson, 1982; Ogier, 1984). They also provide important role model figures for learners and other nurses, and make a significant contribution to the work setting and organisational climate (Fretwell, 1982; Choppin, 1983; Pembrey, 1987). In addition, Lelean (1973) noted how this group played a key role in the collection and dissemination of information to nurses in clinical settings. In practice, they hold a pivotal position, with the power and influence that goes with it. Thus a sample of 25 nurses of sister/charge nurse grade was selected.

A range of clinical areas was selected to include nurses from general, psychiatric, paediatric and midwifery settings. In addition, some of the sample worked in the community while others worked in hospitals. The sampling method employed is known as 'strategic informant sampling' (Smith, 1981); it allows the researcher to tap persons who are well informed about the social setting being investigated. It is usual to select individuals who occupy leadership roles within the organisation.

The sampling procedure was initiated in a number of different ways, first through a 'snowball' method in which those individuals who were contacted at the outset provided the name of one other person for the sample (Coleman, 1958). On several occasions, respondents were asked to recommend other people with different views and perspectives on the topic. Second, there was an expert choice method where senior nurse managers provided the researcher (PM) with the names of individuals in the organisation.

However, this sampling technique has a number of limitations. By selecting those informants occupying key roles – the ward sister/charge nurse group – within the organisation, it omits other trained nurses, both registered and enrolled, and students in training. Similarly, other groups, such as nurse helpers, relatives and especially patients, may well have alternative views of caring.

❏ Setting up the interviews

Informants were contacted initially by phone, and this was followed up by visits to the informants in their working environment. At this time, details about the project and the repertory grid format (devoid of technical language) were given. Confidentiality was assured. The researcher emphasised that the procedure was not a test and that there were no right or wrong answers, only views and opinions. A list of role titles (elements) to be used at the later meeting was also provided. These were:

1. a caring nurse
2. an uncaring nurse
3. the most caring person I know
4. the least caring person I know
5. a person I care a lot for
6. a person I don't care much for
7. myself as a carer, and
8. how I would like to be as a carer (ideal self).

These element role titles were chosen to be representative of the area of inquiry, namely that of how carers construe caring. The informants were asked to identify and match real people to these in their own time. They were instructed to write down only people's initials as it was not necessary for the researcher to know who these people were. A further condition was that they should choose different people for each role element.

The interviews proceeded along the following lines. The researcher asked the informant to think about the individuals they had matched to these role titles in the context of their work as professional carers. Constructs were elicited by a self-identification method (Fransella and Bannister, 1977). This required the informant to consider the 'myself as a carer' element with each of the others in turn. The researcher then asked the informant to suggest important 'likenesses' or 'differences' between these two people. Having conveyed this characteristic to the researcher, the informant was then asked to describe what the opposite of this characteristic meant to them personally.

The same procedure was used for elements 1–6. Element number 8 (ideal self) was examined on two occasions as it was felt to be an important role element for looking at potentially important characteristics. The procedure ensured that each informant produced a repertory grid which had eight elements and eight constructs.

Most of the nurses who took part in the research found the administration of the grid to be an unusual task, but they quickly adapted to it and completed it without difficulty. The constructs which were produced ranged from single words to sentences, some individuals finding it easy to describe differences or likenesses in one word, others appearing happier to use sentences. The researcher's task was one of facilitation (asking for likenesses or differences, sorting the elements in sequence and recording construct labels). When an informant provided several ideas all at once, the researcher referred these back to the informant for clarification.

After the informant had elicited a set of eight constructs, they were asked to rate the eight elements along the construct dimensions produced, using a 7-point rating scale. In this way, it was possible to explore any discrepancies between the 'self' and 'ideal self' elements (Morrison, 1989a).

■ Analysing the interviews

There are basically two approaches to the problem of analysing repertory grid data, and these have been outlined by Bannister and Mair (1968). One approach involves looking at the structure of the data, while the other involves focusing on the content of the constructs which have been elicited from the informant. Although both approaches have been used in the present study, only the content analysis of the construct will be discussed here, while the structural relationships will be dealt with in the next chapter. Figure 2.1 provides an example of a completed grid. Note the way in which the elements and constructs are laid out in the grid.

Content analysis was used to gain some understanding of the concept of caring represented in the grid data for this group of nurses. A number of other studies have also reported the use of content analysis to analyse grid data, for example in a study of personal relationships (Duck, 1973) and in a study to evaluate training practices in social work (Lifshitz, 1974). Landfield (1971) also used a form of content analysis in a study of psychotherapy, while Neimeyer *et al.* (1984) described a content analysis technique for classifying constructs about death. Honess (1985) has argued that the analysis of content or themes is just as important as structural relationships in grid data but that many of the research reports have ignored the significance of content.

The content analysis procedure outlined by Stewart and Stewart (1981) was used to analyse the 200 constructs collected. Key content areas were identified by the researcher, and individual constructs were then allocated to each of these categories. Each of the constructs (both poles) was written on a small card and sorted by the researcher into homogenous content areas or categories. The categories were then labelled according to type of content. A small number of colleagues were asked to check the match between the content type and the label supplied by the researcher. They were also invited to offer alternative labels if they so wished. This resulted in one new category being generated and a minor revision of two of the other labels. Table 2.3 shows the categories which emerged from this procedure.

CONSTRUCTS								ELEMENTS
More qualified	Dedicated	Nervous	Approachable	Disinterested	Efficient	Disorganised	Conscientious	
3	3	5	1	7	1	2	1	A caring nurse
4	4	4	3	4	3	3	4	An uncaring nurse
4	4	4	4	4	1	7	1	The most caring person I know
4	7	1	5	4	2	5	1	The least caring person I know
2	6	3	1	6	2	2	4	A person I care a lot for
4	4	1	4	7	1	7	2	A person I don't care much for
4	4	4	1	6	2	7	1	Myself as a carer
1	1	7	1	7	1	7	1	How I would like to be as a carer (ideal self)
Less qualified	Lacks dedication	Calm	Unapproachable	Interested	Inefficient	Organised	Unfeeling	

Figure 2.1 An example of one complete repertory grid which shows the elements, the elicited constructs and the rating of the elements on each of the constructs. '1' indicates that the top of the construct applies, whereas '7' indicates that the bottom does.

Table 2.3   The seven-category scheme

Category	Number of constructs	Percentage
Personal qualities	78	39.0
Clinical work style	39	19.5
Interpersonal approach	35	17.5
Level of motivation	21	10.5
Concern for others	14	7.0
Use of time	9	4.5
Attitudes	4	2.0
Totals	200	100

The constructs were all then allocated to the category labels. A small number of constructs were marked to indicate to the researcher their category allocation, and some helpful colleagues were asked to sort these into the category framework.

In addition, three of the informants were also invited to re-examine their own constructs in the light of the category scheme developed and to consider the category framework as whole. This procedure helped the researcher to check the adequacy of the descriptive framework (Ashworth, 1987). Small revisions to the scheme were made at this point.

❏ Findings

The seven-category framework presented in Table 2.3 shows the proportion of constructs assigned to each of the categories. It is notable that these proportions vary considerably. For example, 'personal qualities' accounted for 39 per cent of the construct pool, while 'attitudes' accounted for only 2 per cent. The type of category, too, was found to be diverse, ranging from personal qualities attributed to individuals, to how they work in the clinical field and how they interact with others, and included constructs about people's level of motivation, their concern for others, their use of time and their attitudes. Some examples of the categories and the types of construct from which they were developed can be seen in Figures 2.2–2.8.

CARING	UNCARING
Kind	Unkind
Knowledgeable	Not knowledgeable
Helpful	Unhelpful
Genuine	False

Figure 2.2   Personal qualities (constructs used to attribute particular qualities to individuals).

CARING	UNCARING
Treats everyone as an individual	Works like a production line
Skillful nurse	Unskillful nurse
Reliable	Unreliable
Explains treatment and care adequately to patients	Ignores psychological needs of patients

Figure 2.3   Clinical work style (constructs which refer to the way people work in clinical settings).

CARING	UNCARING
Approachable	Unapproachable
Sensitive approach	Thoughtless approach
Listens to people	Doesn't listen
Empathic	Lacks empathy

Figure 2.4   Interpersonal approach (constructs dealing with the way people act in relation to others).

CARING	UNCARING
Highly motivated	Unmotivated
Dynamic	Apathetic
Nothing is too much trouble	Only does what is needed
Conscientious	Negligent

Figure 2.5   Level of motivation (constructs which refer to a person's degree of commitment).

CARING	UNCARING
Puts others before self	Selfish
Gives freely of self	Selfish (egocentric)
Concerned for people	Disinterested in people's welfare
Aware of others	Lacks awareness of others

Figure 2.6   Concern for others (constructs which emphasise unselfishness).

CARING	UNCARING
Always has time for people	Pretends to be busy
Has time for supporting relationships	Lacks time for supporting relationships
Always has time to talk to people	Always has something else to do
Would like to be able to make more time to listen	Pressurised into doing other things

Figure 2.7   Use of time (constructs which focus on how people utilise available time).

CARING	UNCARING
Consistent in attitudes	Inconsistent in attitudes
Easy attitude towards work	Flippant attitude
Down to earth attitude	Condescending attitude
Professional attitude	Lets personal problems intefere with work

Figure 2.8   Attitudes (constructs which refer to particular attitudes).

❏ Discussion of the findings

The framework described above gives a detailed picture of how this group of experienced nurses perceived caring in practice. It provides a British perspective based on qualitative data and is grounded in the views of practising nurses rather than theorists or nurse educators. The categories which emerged from the interviews enable us to look closely at what it means to care for a patient as a professional nurse and as a person. Perhaps one of the most surprising things to emerge was that very few constructs relating to physical care emerged but that a great many could be referred to, in a general sense, as 'psychological'. This point alone suggests the need for further research since nursing is also very much a 'doing' profession. We can, however, suggest some plausible reasons why this should be the case.

The psychological orientation in the constructs produced may be accepted at face value as a snapshot of this group's perception of caring. This account lends support to the view of caring as a particular 'attitude' and provides us with many details of the specific dimensions involved.

A second possible explanation is that it resulted from a limitation of the sample chosen for interview. Since all nurses of charge nurse grade have an important managerial function which ensures that they generally have fewer opportunities to provide bedside nursing care, they have less time available in their work for providing direct care to the patient. Their role, then, may colour their perceptions about caring in nursing.

It is also possible to draw up a comparison between this sample of nurses occupying leadership roles within the organisation and what Taylor and Bogdan (1984) call the 'institutional standard bearers' (see also Goffman, 1961 for a discussion of the staff world). These are the important individuals who stage-manage the impressions of institutions which visitors and outsiders acquire during time spent visiting them. In this sense, informants may have provided data reflecting the current emphasis on psychological needs, to convey a particular storyline to an outside researcher. This picture may not include other relevant dimensions of caring.

However, the large proportion of constructs classed as 'personal qualities' is also rather surprising. While all the sample were highly trained and experienced nurses, their perceptions of caring suggest that it may be a process which has very little to do with training and experience but a lot more to do with the *personal traits* and characteristics which individuals bring with them into the field of nursing.

❏ The caring nurse: an ideal profile

If we assume that the synthesis of these varied categories conveys many of the essential traits of caring in nursing practice, it is possible to develop an ideal picture of a caring nurse. This can be done by combining the most frequently used constructs (caring pole) into a character profile. To do this, only those constructs mentioned on more than two occasions were considered; these have been organised hierarchically so that the most frequently used constructs are listed first. The 'attitudes' category is the weakest in the sense that it is based on only four constructs.

Note, however, that this composite description depicts an ideal type and that, as such, it would be difficult for a nurse in clinical practice to meet these high standards all the time. However, it is not intended to be a prescriptive set of standards. It is offered instead as a description of the way in which some experienced nurses in the UK perceive the nature of caring in a professional context. The ideal profile is as follows:

- *Personal qualities:* the caring nurse is seen to possess a wide range of qualities. He or she is kind, genuine, knowledgeable, patient and calm, has a sense of humour, is helpful, honest, relaxed, assertive, compassionate, considerate, experienced and flexible, has a pleasant disposition, and is tolerant and understanding.
- *Clinical work style:* in work settings, the caring nurse is seen to treat people/patients as individuals and tries to identify patient needs. He or she is organised, puts the patient first and is reliable and skillful.
- *Interpersonal approach:* in his or her relationships with others, the caring nurse is seen to be empathic and approachable, and listens to

people. The approach is sensitive, he or she is easy to get on with and polite, and communicates well with other people.

- *Level of motivation:* the caring nurse is seen to be very interested, conscientious, committed and highly motivated.
- *Concern for others:* the caring nurse is seen to put others before him or herself, and gives freely of him or herself.
- *Use of time:* the caring nurse always has time for people.
- *Attitudes:* the caring nurse is seen to be consistent, down to earth and professional, and has an easy attitude towards work.

❏ Some possible applications in nursing

This small study adds another layer to our attempts to understand what caring is. The findings of this and other studies may have several important applications in other branches of nursing. In theory, it will be possible to use this type of category framework across a range of nursing areas, for example in self- and peer assessment, in organisational appraisals, in the setting of nursing standards, in research programmes, in education and training courses, and perhaps in the selection of candidates for nurse training. However, before this can be done, we must seek out further clarification and empirical support for these descriptive findings. Once that is done useful applications can be developed.

■ Summary

The findings outlined in this study provide many details about nurses' perceptions of the process of caring, using a qualitative application of the repertory grid procedure. These findings reflect some of the shared perceptions of the meaning of caring for this group of nurses. It is interesting to note that the categories of construct found in the construct pool cover the concepts of 'caring' and 'communicating'. They also reflect the 'organisational' context in which these concepts merge and which is the setting where professional caring occurs. However, a great deal of research is needed to describe clearly the nature of a caring relationship. In the next chapter, we examine the notion of the 'caring attitude'.

■ Further reading

Ashworth, P.D. 1995 The meaning of 'participation' in participant observation. *Qualitative Health Research*, **5**(3):366–87.

Brock, S.C. 1995 Narrative and medical genetics: on ethics and therapeutics. *Qualitative Health Research*, **5**(2):150–68.

Engstrom, B. and Nordeson, A. 1995 What neurological patients regard as quality of life. *Journal of Clinical Nursing*, **4**(3):177–83.

Hildingh, C., Fridlund, B. and Segesten, K. 1995 Social support in self-help groups, as experienced by persons having coronary heart disease and their next of kin. *International Journal of Nursing Studies*, **32**(3):224–32.

MacLeod, M.L.P. 1995 What does it mean to be well taught? A hermeneutic course evaluation. *Journal of Nursing Education*, **34**(5):197–203.

Parahoo, K., McGurn, A. and McDonnell, R. 1995 Using research to implement change: the introduction of group activities on a psychiatric unit. *Journal of Clinical Nursing*, **4**(3):195–202.

Rittman, M.R. and Osburn, J. 1995 Interpretive analysis of precepting an unsafe student. *Journal of Nursing Education*, **34**(5):217–21.

Rose, P., Beeby, J. and Parker, D. 1995 Academic rigour in the lived experience of researchers using phenomenological methods in nursing. *Journal of Advanced Nursing*, **21**(6):1123–9.

Rosenal, L. 1995 Exploring the learner's world: critical incident methodology. *Journal of Continuing Education in Nursing*, **26**(3):115–8.

Seed, A. 1995 Conducting a longitudinal study: an unsanitized account. *Journal of Advanced Nursing*, **21**(5):845–52.

Tishelman, C. 1994 Cancer patients' hopes and expectations of nursing practice in Stockholm – patients' descriptions and nursing discourse. *Scandinavian Journal of Caring Sciences*, **8**(4):213–22.

Walsh, K. 1994 Ontology and the nurse–patient relationship in psychiatric nursing. *Australian Journal of Mental Health Nursing*, **3**(4):113–8.

Zemencuk, J., Rogosch, F.A. and Mowbray, C.T. 1995 The seriously mentally ill woman in the role of parent: characteristics, parenting sensitivity, and needs. *Psychosocial Rehabilitation Journal*, **18**(3):77–92.

Chapter Three

The caring attitude

In the last chapter, we discussed some of the literature and research into caring, as perceived by patients and nurses. In addition, we examined a study of nurses' perceptions of caring, using Kelly's personal construct theory and repertory grid technique. We now turn to a more general notion – 'the caring attitude' – which developed out of the study discussed in the last chapter. In this chapter, however, we examine some of the ways in which nurses perceived themselves as professional carers, again using the repertory grid method.

■ The nature of attitudes

Attitudes are an essential part of life. Without attitudes we would not know how to react to some of the things which happen to us on a daily basis, and we would find it very difficult to make decisions. We also spend much time trying to understand and explain human behaviour by referring to some underlying motive, disposition or attitude (Heider, 1958). In social psychology, the term 'attitude' has been the source of much research attempting to explore possible explanations for the things that people do and the ways in which they behave.

Essentially, an attitude is 'a disposition to respond favourably or unfavourably to an object, person, institution, or event' (Ajzen, 1988, p. 4) and which is relatively stable over time. In theory, if we know what a person's attitude is towards, say, the church, we may be able to predict whether or not he goes to church regularly, or whether or not religion influences his day-to-day behaviour.

■ Attitude formation

We acquire attitudes in a number of interesting ways. Learning is a crucial process for attitude formation, in particular the type of learning that occurs when we are socialised by our parents, other family members and friends. The family provides role models for us to emulate, and to do this effectively we must take on board not only the behaviours of key role models but also the attitudes they convey to us.

Furthermore, we also develop our own attitudes from direct exposure to novel experiences. It is only after we have tried out the taste of alcohol or tobacco for ourselves, and experienced their effect on us, that we can form our own attitudes towards these substances. These attitudes may be quite different from those of our parents and elders.

■ The ABC model of attitudes

Although there have been various approaches to the study of attitudes, a common trend has been to think about attitudes in three distinct realms – the affective realm, the behavioural realm and the cognitive realm. This approach is also known as the ABC model of attitudes (Breckler, 1984).

The affective domain centres on the how the person feels about the object, while the behavioural realm refers to the actions of the individual with respect to the given object. The cognitive realm focuses on the information, perceptions and beliefs about the object which are held by the individual. It may be useful to expand on this model with an example.

Suppose we believe that pollution control is necessary for the survival of the planet earth, and we feel very strongly that we should do something about it. One option would be to sell our car, which is a source of pollution – that would certainly cut down on the amount of lead pollution that we contributed to the atmosphere every day. In this case, all the realms of attitude would be in harmony. However, we need a car to get to work each morning. The best solution is for us to convert the engine to run on unleaded fuel. In this way, we can manage to keep the three facets of attitude as closely aligned or consistent as possible.

■ Attitudes and consistency

The issue of consistency has generated a number of theories. Heider (1958) proposed that people have on the whole a preference for consistency and attempt to maintain a state of balance across their system of beliefs, or between what they believe and what they do. If we like someone, we tend to spend time with them. If we dislike someone, we try to avoid being with them. Here the composition of the elements is compatible.

If, however, the situation changes and we have to work with someone we dislike intensely, stress and tension are experienced because the elements are imbalanced. To solve this dilemma, we have to re-appraise our views about that person or resort to another course of action – such as asking to be transferred to another section in the organisation. Only then can the situation return to a state of balance.

Perhaps a more widely known theoretical framework in this field is Festinger's (1957) theory of cognitive dissonance. This approach hinges on the difficulty we feel when we try to hold two inconsistent and conflicting beliefs, or when there is a discrepancy between what we believe and how we behave. In the example cited above, it would be very difficult for us to have strong feelings about lead pollution yet continue to ignore the strength of these feelings each morning as we started up the car for the journey to work. This conflict or dissonance must be resolved in some way, and this is usually achieved by altering attitudes or by adjusting our behaviour.

■ Attitudes in nursing: the example of attitudes to the mentally ill

Most nurses and nursing students care for those with mental health problems at various points during their careers. Mental health and mental illness are potentially emotive issues, so we set out to explore some nursing students' attitudes towards mental illness. There is some evidence to suggest that, when students work with those who are suffering from mental illness, their attitude towards the mentally ill becomes more positive. However, there is also evidence that this positive attitude is often lost when students return to general nursing settings. It may also be noted that attitudes towards certain groups of nursing clients will affect both the levels of care offered to those groups and nurses' career decisions.

We used the Opinions about Mental Illness (OMI) scale devised by Cohen and Struening (1959, 1960). This is a 51-item questionnaire which invites respondents to consider a range of statements about mentally ill people, some of their personal characteristics, the aetiology and treatment of mental illness, and opinions about mental illness itself. A more detailed account of the OMI scale can be found elsewhere (Antonak and Livneh, 1988).

The sample was a convenience one of 115 students on various nursing courses. A convenience sample is one that is available to the researcher and is a form of non-probability sampling. Figure 3.1 illustrates the characteristics of the sample.

SAMPLE CHARACTERISTICS	
Male	10
Female	105
Mean age (years)	22.88
Standard deviation (years)	5.79

Figure 3.1   Characteristics of the student sample (n = 115).

The findings from the completed questionnaires were processed using the Statistical Package for the Social Sciences (SPSS) for Windows. Frequency counts for each of the responses to each of the items were computed. By way of illustration of the findings, we offer a selection of ten responses from the questionnaire in Table 3.1.

Table 3.1   Example of some of the findings from the attitude questionnaire (n = 115)

No. Item	Type	Agree (%)	Unsure/ agree (%)	Unsure/ disagree (%)	Disagree (%)
1. Regardless of how you look at it, patients with severe mental illness are no longer really human	−	2	1	8	104
2. More tax money should be spent on the care and treatment of people with severe mental illness	+	84	26	4	1
3. People who have been patients in a mental hospital will never be their old selves again	−	8	18	27	62
4. People with mental illness should never be treated in the same hospital as people with physical illness	+	10	9	26	70
5. Most patients in mental hospitals are not dangerous	+	59	29	12	15
6. Even though patients in mental hospitals behave in funny ways, it is wrong to laugh at them	+	94	11	6	4
7. Patients in mental hospitals are in many ways like children	−	13	31	21	50
8. Mental illness is an illness like any other	+	68	7	11	29
9. Most women who were once patients in a mental hospital could not be trusted as baby-sitters	−	26	43	35	11
10. Anyone who is in hospital for a mental illness should not be allowed to vote	−	6	12	27	70

Overall, there were positive attitudes in the sample, but note how some respondents felt that people with mental illnesses were no longer really human, that it is not wrong to laugh at people with mental illness or that people in a mental hospital should not be allowed to vote. A surprising number of respondents expressed the view that women who were once in a mental hospital should not be trusted as baby-sitters. It is important to know how people feel about these sorts of issue and to consider how an expressed attitude may influence behaviour. Think for a few moments how you would respond to these statements.

A wide range of attitude measures exists, and many have been developed in the health care context. The interested reader may like to consult some of the following:

Bowling, A. (1995) *Measuring Disease: A review of disease-specific quality of life measurement scales.* Open University Press, Buckingham.

Bowling, A. (1995) *Measuring Health: A reviw of quality of life measurement scales.* Open University Press, Buckingham.

Miller, D.C. (1991) *Handbook of Research Design and Social Measurement*, 5th edn. Sage, London.

Robinson, J.P., Shaver, P.R. and Wrightsman, L.S. (eds) (1991) *Measures of Personality and Social Psychological Attitudes.* Academic Press, London.

■ The link between attitudes and behaviour

So far we have suggested that there is a strong link between our attitudes and our behaviour. Common sense will tell us that this the case. However, the research into the relationship between attitudes and behaviour is less than convincing. Wicker (1969), for example, challenged the assumed close link between attitudes and behaviour when he reviewed the literature on the subject. Most such types of study tend to focus on a mathematical relationship or correlation between attitudes and behaviour, but Wicker found only a very weak correlation between them.

To account for this surprising trend, Wicker suggested that other considerations, such as personal (for example activity levels, other attitudes or motives) or situational (such as the presence of other people, the expected norms) factors may influence the individual. However, since Wicker's account there has been new evidence to suggest that attitudes can predict behaviour under certain conditions (Baron and Byrne, 1987). We now turn our attention to some of these issues.

Some attitudes are very general, while others are very specific. You may have a general attitude against apartheid but not *do* anything to demonstrate consistency between this attitude and your behaviour. On the other hand, you may have a very positive attitude towards healthy food and be sure to always avoid certain foods which have a high fat content. General attitudes may not always produce consistent behaviour, while very specific attitudes nearly always do. The more specific the attitudes being assessed, the greater the accuracy with which behaviour can be predicted.

■ Other factors which influence attitude–behaviour consistency

A number of other factors have also been found to influence the bond between attitudes and behaviour. First, the *strength* of an attitude will be influential. Attitudes that are formed as a result of direct experience tend to be stronger and better predictors of behaviour than attitudes that have been acquired passively (Fazio *et al.*, 1982). Second, when the issues in question have a direct *effect* on the individual's own life and concerns, there is a strengthening of the relationship between attitudes and behaviour (Sivacek and Crano, 1982). Third, attitudes which are more *accessible* to the individual will be more influential (Fazio, 1986). Those attitudes which are strong, and which impinge on the life of the person, will tend to be more accessible. This accessibility will ensure that the attitude is constantly kept in mind and increases the likelihood that it will influence the individual's behaviour.

These factors together emphasise the role of *self-awareness* in understanding how and why we behave as we do in some circumstances and not others. Indeed, some studies have shown that increased self-awareness can promote greater consistency between attitudes and behaviour (Pryor *et al.*, 1977).

■ Attitudes and helping behaviour

If we can accept from the previous discussion that attitudes do in fact influence our behaviour, we can develop the theme further by focusing on the way in which attitudes affect altruistic, helping and caring behaviour. Indeed, Rajecki (1982) has argued that attitudes play a *crucial role* in altruistic and helping behaviour. He suggests that a number of important attitudinal processes may be at work to promote this type of behaviour.

The way in which we decide whether or not a person is *deserving* of help for example, or whether or not we perceive ourselves to be helping and caring individuals, will influence our behaviour. These processes may be understood by reference to attribution theory, which we mentioned in the last chapter, as we are constantly having to decide who is and who is not a deserving case, and we also have perceptions about ourselves as professional carers.

In addition, normative influences from within the context in which care is given, whether they are personally or socially determined, direct us to help or steer clear of a situation. These influences have been observed across a range of clinical nursing settings, including general surgery (Knight and Field, 1981), accident and emergency units (Jeffrey, 1979) and psychiatric nursing (Kelly and May, 1982).

■ The caring attitude

In Griffin's (1983) descriptive analysis of caring which we discussed in Chapter 1, we noted that caring was essentially an interpersonal process. The role of the nurse is to carry out certain activities specific to the role of the nurse in a manner which conveys some feeling to the patient or client. Griffin suggests that 'liking' and 'compassion' may be important facets of the nurse's attitude.

■ Developing a caring attitude scale

This section is an extension of the study described in the previous chapter, so few of the procedural details need to be recounted here. You will recall, however, that we interviewed 25 nurses of charge nurse grade and that the interviews were structured using Kelly's personal construct theory and repertory grid technique (Kelly, 1955).

Each of the nurses produced eight bipolar constructs and then rated eight elements, including a 'myself as a carer' element and an 'ideal self as a carer' element, using a 7-point rating scale. By calculating a simple difference score (Bannister and Mair, 1968; Honey, 1979; Easterby-Smith, 1981) between the 'self' and 'ideal self', it is possible to measure the degree of discrepancy between these two elements. We assume that any observed differences between the two sets of scores indicate the need for personal change, or some sort of inner conflict. Figure 3.2 is an example of how the 'myself as a carer' element was rated for one of the informants.

All of the informants were asked to rate each of the eight elements in turn, along their own set of constructs, by placing a tick at the appropriate point on the scale. These straightforward responses could be easily converted into numerical values at a later date. The two most important elements were the 'myself as a carer' and 'how I would like to be as a carer (ideal self)' because they enabled us to explore people's perceptions of themselves as carers.

MYSELF AS A CARER

Safe	✔ – – – – – –	Dangerous
Selfish	– – – – ✔ – –	Gives freely of themselves
Compassionate	– ✔ – – – – –	Does not see others' needs
Lacks awareness	– – – ✔ – – –	Overprotective
Empathic	– – ✔ – – – –	Lacks sensitivity
Insecure	– – – – ✔ – –	Mature
Tolerant	– – ✔ – – – –	Intolerant
Kind	– ✔ – – – – –	Disinterested

Figure 3.2 Example of the type of rating scale used for each informant.

However, the use of a self-rating technique carried certain risks (Crowne and Marlowe, 1964). Could the informants be relied upon to report their self-perceptions honestly when some of the constructs were so value laden? To get around this potential problem, certain strategies were used. These included, for example, emphasising the importance of giving honest answers, developing a comfortable rapport with the informant and ensuring that each informant was fully aware of what was required of him or her from the beginning (Cook and Selltiz, 1973). However, it can be seen from the analysis of these interviews that the procedure does work and that useful insights may be obtained by working along the lines suggested here.

■ Analysis of the grid data

The completed grid for informant number 12 can be seen in Table 3.2. This shows that differences occurred on six of the eight constructs. Only small differences can be seen on four of the constructs (1, 2, 5 and 6), whereas construct 3 shows a marginally bigger difference of 2. The largest discrepancy occurs on construct 7, with a difference of 6. On constructs 4 and 8, no differences surfaced. These differences were added to yield a total difference score of 12. The possible range of scores was 0–48, where 0 signifies no discrepancy between these elements and 48 means that these elements were at opposite ends of the construct pole for all constructs.

The overall picture of difference scores for the group is given in Figure 3.3. While the possible range of scores was 0–48, the actual range observed was 1–20. The average or mean difference score was 10.96. On many of the constructs, small differences were noted, while much larger discrepancies were seen on others. The general finding was that differences emerged for *all 25* informants.

Table 3.2   Grid data for one informant (no. 12), showing elicited constructs, the pattern of rating for the self and ideal self elements, and the total difference score between these two

CONSTRUCTS			ELEMENTS		
			Self	Ideal self	Difference score
1.	Safe	– – – Dangerous	2	1	1
2.	Selfish	– – – Gives freely of themselves	5	6*	1
3.	Compassionate	– – – Does not see others' needs	3	1	2
4.	Lacks awareness	– – – Overprotective	5	5*	0
5.	Empathic	– – – Lacks sensitivity	3	2*	1
6.	Insecure	– – – Mature	6	7	1
7.	Tolerant	– – – Intolerant	7	1	6
8.	Kind	– – – Disinterested	1	1	0
					Total difference score = 12

See p. 59 for explanation.

SUMMARY STATISTICS	
Mean	10.96
Standard deviation	4.52
Range	1–20

Figure 3.3 Summary of difference scores between the 'self as a carer' and 'ideal self as a carer' elements for all informants (n = 25).

■ The self and the ideal self

The approach used here, which entailed asking people to compare 'themselves' with an 'ideal self' image, is not without its problems. The fact that you ask someone to consider an 'ideal self' may influence what informants will tell you. It may lead them to produce views and opinions about caring in nursing practice which they might not normally have considered or perceived as relevant.

Rating both a 'self' and an 'ideal self' along the construct dimensions could also have biased the informants. Since all the informants had prior knowledge of the procedure, this may have suggested to them that they should rate themselves less favourably because they had to rate an 'ideal self' immediately afterwards. One way around this difficulty would be get independent raters, for example other practising nurses or indeed patients, to complete the scale, and to compare both sets of scores. However, such a procedure has its own problems, particularly if you ask patients to evaluate nurses' performance.

If we put these procedural difficulties to one side for the moment, it could be argued that a larger sample of nurses, or indeed other helping and caring professionals, would also highlight discrepancies between the 'self' and 'ideal self' in terms of the caring role. Furthermore, such a finding is perhaps not at all surprising given the inherently difficult and demanding work required from all the helping professions.

Of course, it may well be that it is impossible for nurses and other carers, be they professional or informal, to live up to these ideal levels. However, if we assume that the role discrepancies outlined above are an important source of personal conflict and stress, it is interesting to note that a number of psychological theories have stressed the way in which people struggle to minimise conflict of this nature.

The theory of self-consistency outlined by Lecky (1961) explores how the individual changes to avoid tension and contradictions. Similarly, Festinger's theory of cognitive dissonance, which we mentioned earlier, describes how people try to reduce the feelings of discomfort experienced when they are confronted with situations contrary to their own beliefs and views of the world (Festinger, 1957). Similarly, Rogers (1965) discussed how one of the goals of psychotherapy was to enable the 'self' and 'ideal self' to become more compatible.

If nurses also try to reduce the level of 'inconsistency' in themselves, the method of comparing 'self' and 'ideal self' may prove to be a very useful way to explore self-perceptions and to judge the degree and direction of any changes. In addition, a programme of self-assessment could easily be set up to take account of any other events or happenings at the same time. In this way, we may be able to learn a lot more about nurses' perceptions of themselves as carers and about how different aspects of their work influence their self-perceptions.

■ Why do these discrepancies exist?

If the work of the nurse is to care for people, and this is what she has been trained to do, why should these discrepancies occur so consistently? A number of possible explanations may be suggested. First, the nurses who took part in the study may have set very unrealistic expectations for themselves. This would make it impossible for them to live up to their personal standards. Second, the discrepancies may in fact be the result of inappropriate or inadequate training for the job which they now do. The group may lack the knowledge and skills necessary to fulfil their caring role in the desired manner. Third, it is possible that the system of values which can be found within the 'organisational culture' (Schein, 1984) may be quite unlike the values cherished by the individual nurses working in the organisation. So technical competence may be valued more than interpersonal (caring) competence within the organisation, and this influences the way in which the nurses perceive themselves. One the one hand, nurses feel the need to develop close caring relationships with patients and clients. On the other hand, the notions of efficiency and effectiveness are so prevalent within the institution that the nurse has little choice but to toe the line and go along with the dominant ethos of the organisation.

There are other potential reasons which might help us to account for these findings, but they must remain, for the moment, speculative suggestions. Much more research needs to done before more detailed explanations can be put forward.

■ The personal cost of caring

However, one other possible explanation of the discrepancies found between the 'self as a carer' and 'ideal self' elements must be considered. It was noted that when the informants were asked to rate all eight elements on the construct dimensions, a particular pattern of rating emerged in many of the interviews. Closer inspection showed that it emphasised the *personal cost of caring for the carer*. This can be clearly seen in Figure 3.3.

You can see in Table 3.2 that three of the construct ratings for the 'ideal self' are marked with an asterisk. It was expected that the 'ideal self' element would be rated on the extremes of all the construct dimensions, but, as can be seen, this did not occur for constructs 2, 4 and 5. When this happened in the interview, the informant was asked why she rated the 'ideal self' in this way. In this case, the nurse said that to place herself on these extremes of the construct dimensions might 'result in me being physically and emotionally drained'. This informant nurse had grave doubts about *always* 'giving freely of oneself,' being 'overprotective' and being 'empathic'.

Out of a total of 25 interviews, 12 of the informants completed the rating procedure in the same way. Several other comments were recorded to justify this pattern of rating, including the following: 'may result in burnout', 'stress', 'other priorities in the caring process' and 'unhealthy for both the carer and the cared-for person'. This would support the general assertion that the work of the nurse is intrinsically 'stressful' (Marshall, 1980), and, like other professions with a client-centred emphasis, nurses are likely to experience 'burnout' (Pines *et al.*, 1981).

■ Other explanations

The unexpected rating can be explained by focusing on changes in the ways nurses perceive their caring role. It is possible, and indeed likely, that these nurses are taking active steps to promote *independence* among patients. If we keep this in mind, we are able to re-interpret some of the verbatim explanations provided by informants to account for the surprising pattern of ratings. In particular, 'other priorities in the caring process' and 'unhealthy for both the carer and the cared-for person', may be indicating, albeit implicitly, the nurses' appreciation of the need to promote greater patient independence.

The findings in general do share similarities with those of other studies, in that they stress the demands placed upon carers. Others have reported that caring for people is both *physically* and *emotionally* exhausting. In community settings, Hirschfeld (1983) and Goodman (1986) have described the immense strain that caregivers experience, whereas others (Hyde, 1976; Llewelyn, 1984, 1989) have reflected on the potentially harmful effects of caring nurse–patient relationships.

Hyde (1976) stresses the need to care for ourselves. In this way our potential for caring for others is positively enhanced. Llewelyn (1984, 1989) argues that while close interpersonal (caring) relationships are more demanding, they are also more effective and offer opportunities for personal growth and development. This emphasis can also be found in Mayeroff's descriptive account of the caring process (Mayeroff, 1972).

■ How would you rate yourself as a carer?

In the final section of this chapter, we have drawn up a general grid to allow you to rate yourself as a carer on some of the constructs which were generated from the research described in this book. You may, in fact, have your own ideas about what it means to care for another person as a nurse and as a person and think that some of the constructs do not apply well to you. That's fine. There will always be this sort of individual variability where human beings are concerned.

	ELEMENTS	
Kind	– – – – – –	Unkind
Patient	– – – – – –	Impatient
Unhelpful	– – – – – –	Helpful
Honest	– – – – – –	Untrustworthy
Tolerant	– – – – – –	Intolerant
Disorganised	– – – – – –	Organised
Treats people as individuals	– – – – – –	Ignores individual needs
Not empathic	– – – – – –	Empathic
Unapproachable	– – – – – –	Approachable
Listens	– – – – – –	Does not listen
Insensitive	– – – – – –	Sensitive
Genuine	– – – – – –	False
Knowledgeable	– – – – – –	Not knowledgeable
Highly motivated	– – – – – –	Lacks motivation
Selfish	– – – – – –	Unselfish
Has time for people	– – – – – –	Lacks time for people

Figure 3.4   The caring grid.

We suggest that you take a pencil and paper and rate yourself on the grid shown in Figure 3.4. Think about yourself as you are at present in a working context with patients or clients, and then consider yourself in terms of each construct in turn. Do not spend too much time thinking about your response on each construct. Just tick the point on the construct scale which reflects your views. For example, if you feel that are *always* kind, then you might tick the dash closest to the word 'kind'. If on the other hand you feel that you are sometimes kind and at other times unkind in your relationships with patients, you might feel that it is more accurate to tick the midpoint in the scale. Rate yourself on all constructs and then join each point to form a line from top to bottom.

Now rate how you think your ideal self would be, but this time *circle* the point which reflects your views. Join the circles together with a line from top to bottom. Are the two lines close together or far apart? If the lines are far apart, this suggests a wide discrepancy between yourself as a carer and your ideal self as a carer. We think that most people will observe some discrepancies. Why do you think this is the case? Are there particular aspects of your work at the moment which may be influential and have not been discussed above? Discuss your rating with colleagues.

■ Summary

This chapter has discussed the nature of an attitude and has described some of the important issues related to attitudes and attitude research. The concept of the 'caring attitude' was introduced and described. We also discussed some of the research findings which looked at nurses' perceptions of themselves as carers. Discrepancies between the nurses' perceptions of the 'self' and 'ideal self' were examined, and possible explanations for these discrepancies were addressed.

■ Further reading

Diamond, P. and Thompson, M. 1985 Using personal construct theory to assess a midwives' refresher course: students' constructions (perceptions) of their professional roles. *Australian Journal of Advanced Nursing*, **2**(4):24–6, 28–35.

Fox, J., Scaman, H. and Wilmot, S. 1993 Caring: a new framework for analysis. *British Journal of Nursing*, **2**(20):1008–11.

Franks, V., Watts, M. and Fabricius, J. 1994 Interpersonal learning in groups: an investigation. *Journal of Advanced Nursing*, **20**(6):1162–9.

Swanwick, M. and Barlow, S. 1994 How should we define the caring role? Broadening the parameters of the concept of care. *Professional Nurse*, **9**(8):554, 556–9.

Chapter Four

Caring for patients

The findings reported in earlier chapters helped to draw up a picture of caring in nursing from the nurse's point of view, but these findings are limited by the methods chosen to carry out the interviews with nurses. On the one hand, the repertory grid provided a great deal of structure and was easy to analyse. On the other hand, use of the grid restricted the types of question we could ask and the richness of the data that were collected. In this chapter, we describe the results of more qualitative study of nurses' experiences of caring for patients in a professional context. In the next, we explore the patients' perspective.

■ A phenomenological approach to understanding nurses' experiences

The phenomenological approach has gradually gained wider acceptance in the field of qualitative health research. There are several advocates of the approach as it applies to studies in nursing (see for example Omery, 1983; Watson, 1985; Drew, 1986; Swanson-Kauffmann and Schonwald, 1988; Holmes, 1990). The approach is very different from the traditional approach employed in social science research. Phenomenology is an attempt to really get to know how another person is experiencing his or her world, and has the potential to be especially useful in professional helping and caring relationships.

Kestenbaum (1982a) argued a case for the use of existential phenomenology in health care research on the grounds that it provided a powerful set of techniques for exploring patient and professional viewpoints which could be used in practice. A further advantage of the phenomenological perspective is that it can foster the development of a diverse range of understandings of illness, health and health care workers (Kestenbaum, 1982b).

An in-depth discussion of the underlying theory and associated approaches to interviewing and analysis may be found elsewhere (see for example Giorgi, 1970; Valle *et al.*, 1989; Spinelli, 1989), while details about the specific approach used to guide the study referred to in this and the next chapter have been discussed in Morrison (1991, 1992, 1994).

■ The interviews with nurses

The main aim of this component of the study was to explore in depth some nurses' experiences of caring for patients at work. A purposive sample of 10 nurses (informants) from medical, surgical and psychiatric wards were asked to talk about their experiences of 'caring for patients'. The interviews were guided by a small set of questions that focused on *what* the nurses did for patients and *how* they did their work. Each nurse was asked to recount a specific patient they cared for and to describe the account in great detail.

All the nurses in the study worked in a large teaching hospital and held different positions in the organisation – charge nurse, staff nurse, state enrolled nurse, student and nursing assistant. Both male and female nurses took part. The interviews were tape-recorded and later transcribed word for word. Most of the interviews were carried out in or around a practical ward setting – a side ward or examination room was usually available which was quiet enough and private enough for an interview. This procedure produced a very detailed picture of the nurses' experiences. The remainder of this chapter outlines a shortened and more readable account of the main findings. Some direct quotations are included to give the reader a flavour of the interviews. Note how this approach has produced findings that are very different from those of the earlier repertory grid studies.

❏ Summary of analysis procedure

The procedure used to analyse these interviews and those described in the following chapter have been described elsewhere, but it may be helpful to provide here a brief overview of the principal stages in that analysis (Figure 4.1).

■ The main themes in the nurses' interviews

The findings from the interviews with nursing staff are presented in the form of nine general themes which captured the nurses' experiences of 'caring for patients' in hospital. The general themes are presented with

1. A focused interview with each informant was taped and initially analysed on the same day. A verbatim transcript of the interview was completed at a later date and divided into natural meaning units.
2. The transcribed text was restated in the third person and reorganised into distinct content areas. These content areas were given initial labels.
3. The central themes to emerge from the interview which communicated the informant's perceptions about the experience of caring or being cared for were outlined.
4. A comparison of themes was made across interviews in an effort to discover common themes. In addition the findings of the nursing group and the patient group were compared. A general re-examination of the literature related to the research was undertaken so that the findings could be located within a particular research context.

Figure 4.1 Summary of the principal stages in the interview analysis.

supporting sub-themes underneath each main heading. Occasionally a third level of sub-heading has been used to highlight very fine discriminations in the informants' accounts. These reflect many of the important themes that characterise the nurses' experience of caring for patients in hospital. The names of the nurses involved in the study have been changed. The main themes were:

1. hopelessly dependent cases
2. felt impact of the patient's dreadful situation
3. did their best for patients
4. calculated emotional involvement with patients
5. constant awareness of the stressful nature of the work
6. superficial preparation for the job
7. constrained by the ward environment
8. coped with a demanding and uncertain role
9. personal benefits derived from caring for others.

❏ Theme 1: Hopelessly dependent cases

A most striking aspect of the nurses' accounts was the type of case almost all staff recalled and described in detail. The term 'hopelessly dependent cases' captures the type of patient who elicited caring responses in these nurses.

Terminally ill and frightened
Jeff looked after a young intelligent lady with a family:

She got to the stage of her illness where she was very frightened, extremely frightened. That's why she was admitted and she didn't really know what to expect. She had terminal cancer...

She wanted to know everything about the treatment and the side-effects. She was worried about what her husband would do after her death and about the fact that her son became very frightened when her hair started to fall out because of the treatment.

Faced a lonely and inevitable death
Another young staff nurse, Emma, looked after a long-stay patient who was dying of cancer and waiting for a hospice place. Emma felt that the patient was 'alone' even though she shared a four-bedded room with other patients.

Deserving of care
Steve looked after a 26-year-old patient who was very depressed and was admitted after an overdose of insulin. Initially, the patient needed a lot of physical care, was in a dreadful state and had had a low opinion of himself:

I think we struck a chord because he was so obviously depressed, it was just an illness and he didn't do anything to deserve it...

He was deserving of care and Steve liked him because he was a trier.

Depressed and dependent
Three of the staff focused on one particular patient. Trudy got to know another long-stay patient who became very dependent and could not or would not do anything for herself. Trish and Aine nursed this same depressed lady. The patient had been rejected and lost her dignity, and she was difficult to communicate with and incontinent. Trish felt that the patient's family should have been more involved, but unfortunately her husband did not want to spend money on her. Trish really liked this patient, independent of her being so helpless.

Faced traumatic surgery alone
Mona nursed an elderly lady who suddenly became ill and needed heart surgery while her husband was abroad. Her relatives could not visit her, and she was frail, helpless, dependent and very frightened.

Chronic disability and depression
Another nurse, Ruth, looked after an elderly diabetic patient who had had both legs amputated and who eventually died after severe complications. The patient's family could not cope, so the patient needed total care, especially when she was acutely depressed. She also needed a lot of psycholog-

ical support. In spite of her disabilities, the patient was a real trier, a personality on the ward.

Needed a life-saving heart transplant

Dan looked after a family man in his forties with a severe cardiac condition brought on by alcoholism who needed a heart transplant to save his life. The prognosis was poor and the patient knew this. He was placed on the waiting list for a transplant but deteriorated suddenly and died. The patient was not a complainer, but a nice person. At the end, he was nursed alone in a single cubicle.

Dependent and starved of attention

Cath, a student nurse, looked after an elderly patient with breathing difficulties who was very distressed and dependent. He did not receive much attention from the permanent staff:

> He was very dependent on me and other nurses... I felt he was totally starved of staff attention...

❏   Theme 2: Felt impact of the patient's dreadful situation

The second major theme to emerge reflects how the staff *felt* about the patients' circumstances – some facing inevitable death, severe pain or chronic disease and disability. The nurses were moved by the situations the patients had to deal with.

Felt sorry

Nearly all the nurses 'felt sorry' for the patients they cared for. For example, Dan felt sorry for one patient because of the lack of hope of improvement:

> I don't know really, I felt sorry for him in a way but not in the way you'd see something on the telly. I think mostly I felt sad because I would probably have known sooner than him that we weren't going to be able to do anything for him...

Helpless or able to help

Cath and Mona felt pretty helpless. Cath noted that she was:

> feeling quite helpless about it... like not being able to do things that I'd want to do about it, and do things that I thought were appropriate...

Aine felt that she could do nothing more for the patient because everything possible had been done. The nurses were moved by a feeling of being able to help their patients in spite of the awful circumstances in which the patients found themselves. Jeff felt that he could do a lot for the frightened patient in his care, as did Steve, Trish and Dan.

Wanted to give

Cath felt very emotional about caring for her patient because he was in such obvious distress. In general, she just 'felt for patients', and this triggered a caring response:

> the emotion of feeling wanting to make it all right. I wanted to give something of myself though I don't know which category it goes in, it's still a feeling of wanting to make it all right for somebody else but being prepared to give out to somebody else...

Felt anger and revulsion

While Trish felt sorry for her patient, she also felt angry because of the lack of progress and the crippling effects of illness on patients generally: anybody could end up just like this depressed patient. Although Trish realised that looking after the patient's basic needs was important, she still felt revulsion when she had to clean up the patient's mess for the first time:

> the thing was I just talked myself into thinking it was something else, now I find it quite easy but that was the first time I had to clean anybody, you see this could be coming into it... she was the first real patient then, that I did everything for but I did feel revulsion the first time...

Worried and concerned about the patient

One of the patients Emma looked after reminded her of her mother who was of similar age. Emma was concerned that the patient was someone's mother and could have been her own. She worried about the patient, who became part of her life, and looking after the patient raised questions about dying, which she found difficult to face; looking after the patient raised many 'why' questions for her.

Sense of loss and sadness

The death or transfer of patients provoked a feeling of sadness or loss in several nurses. Aine felt an acute sense of loss when the distraught patient she cared for was transferred to another ward where her prospects were not good. Ruth's patient was being prepared for discharge when she died suddenly:

> I certainly felt very sad the day she died 'cause I came back after days off and the whole ward was just like... nothing... It was as quiet as anything and you simply knew something had happened, and I really

felt very very sad… we were all pretty choked up… we were just getting plans for home ready, suddenly it was all gone and that was it.

The ward was not the same after the patient had died and it was sad to look back. Jeff was also very upset by this death and found it was difficult to handle. On the day she died, Jeff had been called back to the ward to see her, and he felt guilty because he was not with her when she died.

Not being able to follow up patients was disruptive to the continuity of care. Emma really wanted to see her patient after she had gone to the hospice but could not.

❏ Theme 3: Did their best for patients

This general theme summarises how the nurses perceived the effectiveness of the way in which they actually cared for the patients.

Spent time with the patient
An important first step in caring for patients was the nurses' ability to spend time with individuals. The level of physical care needed by the patients tended to influence the amount of time the nurses actually spent with them. Jeff sat with his patient and got to know the family well. Cath spent a lot of time giving basic care, such as feeding him, and Trudy spent every spare moment with him. However, spending a large amount of time caring for one particular patient often posed problems for the staff. Aine and other staff, for example, realised how much time they were giving to one patient, and this meant that other patients may have been neglected.

Helped the patient to cope
The nurses helped the patients to cope with their situations in various ways.

Undemanding acceptance
Steve helped his patient to cope with low self-esteem, but not by just telling him to 'cheer up'. He realised that the patient was very alone and frail so he did not make demands on him and tried not to frighten him. Aine accepted her patient but not the patient's behaviour.

Tried to provide a therapeutic environment
Steve tried to provide an environment conducive to psychiatric improvement in an unstructured way. He needed an imaginative approach to interact with his psychotic patient.

Gave personalised and sensitive care

This theme showed up in a range of ways. Emma found herself constantly aware of her patient's needs throughout the day. She put things within reach of the patient to reduce her boredom, made sure she had a drink, something to read and her glasses, and found a vase for her flowers. She wanted to help the patient by doing the things she could not do for herself.

Treated the patient as a worthy person

Emma cared for her as a person and not just a patient – she tried not to treat her like an object on a production line, but wanted to make the patient feel that she mattered. Trish also thought that a caring approach was one that recognised that a patient was first and foremost a person.

Tried to promote independence

The nurses tried to promote independence in patients rather than take over the situation and do everything for them. Some tried to help the patients to help themselves, and involved them in decisions about their care. Trudy tried not to do too much for a patient until it was absolutely necessary.

Recognised the danger of promoting dependence

One of the problems of doing too much for the patients was seen to be the danger of promoting dependence, the key to success being to strike a balance between doing too much and neglecting the patient. The dangers of promoting dependence were recognised by the nurses. However, Trish could not stand by and watch a patient 'starve' because she could not feed herself properly, so it could be hard to draw the line between dependence and the need to promote independence. Aine could not sit and watch the patient doing nothing for herself; she did too much because of a shortage of staff. And Ruth knew that the high level of physical care given may have promoted dependence on the staff.

Paid attention to detail

Another approach used by the nurses was to focus their attention on small but significant aspects of patient care. Cath was acutely aware of things which had relevance for her patient. She took off the oxygen inhaler when it was not needed and put gauze on the mask to prevent soreness. She remembered to put her patient's glasses on and joked with him about his sore feet. However, Cath found that she became upset that many things were not done for the patient by other members of staff when she was not there. Trish made sure that the patient was seated near the window or close to the television. Aine read her patient magazines. Other nurses provided specific examples such as 'take the patient off the ward and to her own home when she asked', and others initiated a programme of toilet training to help deal with an incontinent patient.

Attended to patients' basic needs
Several nurses had to provide a lot of basic nursing care for their patients, including washing, dressing, feeding and lifting them. In a way, caring was demonstrated through managing the patients' basic needs – physical needs took priority.

Physical care helped to develop an empathic response
The practice of providing physical care for patients played an important role in developing an empathic understanding of the patient's situation. In this way, closer relationships with patients were formed. Caring physically provided openings to care for and support the patient emotionally and psychologically. Such intimate physical care offered Emma a way to become more caring.

Empathy was a quality which assumed great importance for the nurses in building close relationships. Jeff was sympathetic towards other people, but he developed a genuine empathy for his patients and built close relationships. Steve was more cautious: he felt that being too empathic could result in the wrong decisions being made.

Optimistic rapport
Another approach employed by the nurses was to adopt an air of unwarranted optimism while in the company of patients. Dan tried to boost his patient's morale, and this lifted his own spirits, although Dan found that he could not be completely honest about the patient's poor chances and uncertain future.

Told the patient not to worry
Although Mona knew her patient's operation was risky, she told the patient not to worry and emphasised the positive aspescts preoperatively. She discouraged the patient from thinking too much about the risks and urged patients generally to think about getting better; they were always very nervous because they were so close to a big operation, and she just wanted to ease their anxiety.

Tried not to let on
Dan tried not to let on to his patient that he 'knew the score' and encouraged him to answer his own questions. He tried not to fuss around the patient too much and wanted to carry on with nursing care in a routine way. He did not want the patient to feel that he was being over-attentive and wondered if he was 'playing it right'. The patient, however, probably knew the prognosis anyway.

Dedicated during working hours only

Steve was dedicated to caring for others, but he reserved this dedication for working hours only: he felt it was not his whole life – he was just a nurse doing a job. Cath felt caring when she was on the ward because that was where it made sense, whereas discussions about patients outside work were boring.

Important interpersonal skills for helping

The nurses reported that several essential skills were needed to care effectively for patients.

Listened attentively

One important skill which Jeff and Dan employed was listening. Jeff did not say much; he 'just listened' attentively to what the patient had to say. Dan said he encouraged his patient to talk about how he felt and offered him a listening ear; he was just there for him to talk to.

Encouraged the patient to talk

Jeff reported that he talked to his patient generally at first and later about death and dying. He got the impression she was glad Jeff could talk about such topics, and she was able to voice her anxieties about dying and her feelings. She knew she was dying and wanted to talk, so Jeff encouraged her to do so. Emma tried to provide an atmosphere of privacy so that her patient felt she could ask for things and was not afraid of Emma.

Gave information

Another aspect of good nursing care was giving information. Jeff tried to keep his patient and her husband informed about what was happening, but he could not answer all her questions. Dan did not have answers for the patient, but he was able to give the patient some factual information about the risks and probabilities.

❑ Theme 4: Calculated emotional involvement with patients

A fourth major theme to emerge focused on the level of emotional involvement that the staff developed with their patients.

Risky emotional involvement

One of the first things to surface here was the recognition that emotional involvement with patients carried some risks, which was widely acknowledged. There was an emotional investment in everything Steve did, and at times he felt too exposed to trust patients. He did not want to be abused and hurt, so he did not invest emotions in patients and run the risk of stress when things went wrong, as some of his colleagues did. Emma also recognised that being involved meant that she could get hurt.

Choosing to be involved

Caring for patients involved making decisions about getting involved with them at some emotional level. For Emma, caring meant being involved and being concerned, which meant that she had to choose to get involved – or not:

> For me there is the internal dimension of choosing to care, to be concerned about people and that they matter to me. This is an internal choice...

Cath, too, was happy to be involved with her patient, while for Aine, caring meant getting involved with patients.

Controlled involvement was more helpful

It was important that any involvement did not get out of control. Cath did not feel that her level of involvement with her patient was out of control, and what she felt was not unreasonable as a professional carer. She had not reached a point where she felt she had given too much of herself. The ward situation controlled Trudy's emotional involvement; she was not supposed to become attached to patients or show much affection for them, although she sometimes did.

Ruth felt the need to have control over her emotions in order to be helpful to patients and their relatives. As a nurse, she had to draw the line and stay in control, although she saw a very fine division between professional caring and being too involved. An empathic understanding helped Ruth not to get caught up in the problems she had to deal with, but she felt that sympathy was unhelpful.

Varied levels of attachment

Although Trish was told not to get too attached to patients, she did become attached and gave a lot of herself to her patients. Generally, she was inclined to become attached to the long-stay patients, which entailed risks. In an acute-care setting, Dan had few opportunities to form attachments. The rapid turnover influenced the way in which patients were perceived and the types of relationship which were formed between the nurses and patients. Dan saw most admissions as 'patients rather than persons'. When Dan did not like someone, he treated them like a 'patient' all the time.

Quickly forgot about patients

One strategy for dealing with over-involvement was to forget about the patients quickly once they had left the ward, as Mona did. She never became too involved with patients, unlike other nurses she knew, because it could be too upsetting when a patient died. Mona was 'hard' and tried to avoid over-involvement – she comforted herself with the knowledge that she did her best for patients.

Unfair expectations of patients

While the risks of involvement for staff were considerable, some of the nurses recognised that the risks for patients were even greater. In a psychiatric setting, Steve expected everything from the patient and recognised how unfair this was:

> Perhaps it is justified because they are the ones who are ill and they're going to get better afterwards, so perhaps they ought to take a risk. I'm not doing it for my health so why should I take a risk. I mean perhaps that is justification, it might not be. I don't know what to do about it.

Difficult to distinguish professional caring from loving

The relationship between caring and loving patients was explored. Although, for some nurses, professional caring relationships did not involve love, Cath saw caring as a part of the process of loving which was a more long-term thing. However, it was not felt necessary for carers to love patients: Mona thought that loving was not appropriate in nursing, except perhaps when looking after children.

❏ Theme 5: Constant awareness of the stressful nature of the work

Another general theme was the stress experienced by staff in their work. Most of the nurses found the work stressful, sources of stress varying considerably.

Constant worry

The lack of a break from the constant worry of the job was felt by a number of nurses. Jeff needed a release valve because he thought about his work 24 hours a day. Emma was stressed because she took her job home with her and found that she could not just switch off at the end of the day. Dan found himself worrying about his patients at home but knew that if he worried too much and could not cope, he might end up not coming to work because it was too much. Mona found it hard when she asked herself if she had done enough for patients.

Wrong attitudes produced stress

The attitude towards work also produced tension in some of the nurses, as shown by Steve, who had the wrong attitude – he had a chip on his shoulder and he took things personally when things went wrong.

Expected abuse

Some nurses who worked on the psychiatric ward shared a similar expectation of abuse from patients. Steve expected no thanks, but only abuse and poor pay. However, he wanted to care and tried not to let his negative expectations influence him too much. Trudy also found it difficult to accept abuse from patients and felt angry. She also knew that, although patients were sometimes nasty, they could not help themselves.

Sending patients back home

One student nurse, Cath, found it particularly upsetting to send patients back into the environment which she knew contributed to their illness, and this also made her feel helpless. She felt stressed and sad because she recognised that many of them were not going to remain well in their own environment:

> you know that they are not going to stay at whatever you've got them to… knowing that they're going home and that a lot of things that sort of precipitated their coming into hospital, I guess they're still going to be there. I think that is partly the never-endingness part of the job… you can't ever whittle it down.

Cath had to accept that there were some things she could not do anything about.

Heightened awareness of personal vulnerability

The incidents described by two of the nurses made them acutely aware of their own vulnerability. Cath found it hard to look at patients and think 'it could be me', while Dan realised how well he was when looking after a dying patient – and how it could have been him. He thought about how the patient's wife must have felt facing the inevitable death of her husband.

Listening to and watching ill people

Having to listen and take on board the pain and suffering of others was also found to be arduous. Cath found it difficult to listen to upsetting things which patients told her, and nursing dying patients was sad enough to make her sometimes cry. It was felt to be very hard to watch people struggling against illness.

Stressful colleagues

Relationships between colleagues also created tension for some. The nearly all-female workforce was a source of stress, the hierarchical system was a burden and some nurses felt intimidated by the unapproachable doctors. Ruth also came into conflict with doctors over what was their responsibility, and she was not prepared to cover up for them. Mona found colleagues a source of stress; sometimes all the girls together were 'bitchy' and could not get along. Ruth found it wearing to watch lazy and uncaring doctors because they sometimes put patients at risk. Dan also found it very stressful to 'chase up' doctors, physiotherapists and pharmacists.

Blamed by the doctors

Mona had to chase up the new doctors and show them what to do, although she felt that some doctors did not care enough to sort out really ill patients and then blamed her when a patient suddenly got worse. She acknowledged that she took the blame for most of the things that went wrong, which was stressful.

Disagreed with doctors about the need for surgery

Ruth questioned the quality of life provided on the ward for one patient because she did not see the point in carrying out a second amputation since the patient was already very ill. After the second operation, the patient went downhill – Ruth felt it would have been better not to have operated, but the medical staff insisted.

Felt unable to challenge established attitudes

As a student, Cath had a different attitude to the qualified staff, whom she felt were often overly critical and judgmental of patients. They were sometimes unsympathetic or even irritated by patients, and Cath found this difficult to handle. Although she did not agree with the more experienced nurses' views on patients, she felt unable to challenge the experienced staff because she lacked confidence.

Did not stir things up

Cath wanted to be able to say what she felt and have it accepted, but she did not want to antagonise staff and get the 'degree students' a bad name. Trudy, a nursing assistant in a psychiatric ward, also had some disagreements with the trained staff but asked herself:

> Do you say something or do you keep quiet because you can't stand a full scale war…?

No time for the students
The relationship that Cath had with the qualified staff was very formal, there being a division between them and the students. It was reported that many students did not look forward to going on the ward because it appeared that staff did not have much time for students generally.

Short student placements
Cath found that working as a student on the ward was stressful because she never really got into it; her time there was too short. However, she felt she learnt a lot quickly by moving from ward to ward.

Never accepted as part of a team of carers
One problem Cath faced as a student was being accepted into the ward team. She felt that she was never accepted like the regular staff, so she had to make a big effort to get to know many new and different people after each move. However, this experience may have a positive side to it as many inexperienced nursing students spend more time with patients because they have not yet become 'team members'.

Observing suicidal patients
In the field of psychiatric nursing, the observation of suicidal patients was identified as being particularly stressful. Trudy experienced extreme stress and panic in such situations:

> You start counting the hours until it's time to go home. When you do go home you're still thinking about it and can't relax. It takes a while to unwind. A lot of the time you feel like I've got to go back to work in so many hours and it's going to start over again... you have to have eyes everywhere...

Difficult relationships with patients
Some of the nurses also found that relationships with 'difficult' patients created tension. Trudy found it wearing when her personal feelings, which she found hard to block out, had to take a backseat in case they interfered with a patient's well-being. Trish experienced stress when she was unable to get through to the patient and communicate in any meaningful way.

Having several patients compete for her attention was draining for Trish, and she sometimes had to ask the patients to be reasonable about the demands they placed on her time. She also sometimes found it difficult when she did not like a particular patient or a patient did not like her. When this happened, she left these patients to other nurses; she realised it was impossible to like everybody.

Mona was stressed by patients who asked her questions and who did not have confidence in her ability:

It all depends on the type of patients you get. You'll have some patients who will question everything that you do and don't have any confidence in you at all. You can get quite worked up.

Aine found it hard when patients unloaded their problems and expected her to have all the answers. It was also difficult to have to listen repeatedly to the same problems. Occasionally, some patients wanted to maintain contact outside the hospital, but Aine needed time away from work.

Shortage of staff increased stress

Aine thought that nurses did not spend enough time with patients because there was a shortage of them. The staff were believed to be under stress because:

> on an acute ward the delivery part of care isn't always the same from day to day...

Lack of positive results

Aine was stressed by a lack of positive results when a particular line of care did not work out and she had to try other approaches to the problem.

Physically and emotionally drained

Ruth found the work psychologically very wearing:

> it can take a lot out of you. If you've got somebody who's physically and mentally, you know, psychologically demanding, and you've gone home some days feeling absolutely drained. You haven't got anything else to give to anybody... you just want to be left alone...

She pushed herself too far and the workload was often formidable. Dan found that not being able to complete what he wanted to do because of changing ward circumstances was hard; the high-dependency patients had to get priority. Heavy workloads were demanding and commonly led to physical and mental exhaustion.

Ways of dealing with stress

In order to be able to continue to care for patients, the nurses had to learn to cope with the routine strains and stresses associated with the role of the nurse. Failure to deal adequately with these could lead many students or even qualified nurses to find alternative employment. A range of possible factors and strategies was identified. Some nurses found that seeing patients recover made the situation more tolerable, whereas others made a conscious effort to get away from the field of work. Emma had to get away and take a break:

I have to get out. When stress levels are very high I feel that I want to withdraw. When you have a difficult incident on the ward I feel like I could make it go away. It's all related to stress. I don't think it's something that you really mean, it's just that you reach the limits of what you can give and I need a break to recharge the batteries.

Jeff tried to keep up to date as a way of relieving stress, as it enabled him to give out accurate information. Steve, on the other hand, felt that most people had a limit to their ability to care. He drew the line when his work interfered with his personal life or when patients were too demanding emotionally.

Personal relationships were sustaining
Personal relationships were also found to be helpful. Cath found that her relationships outside work helped to sustain her; however, giving too much to these relationships sometimes limited what she could do in work.

Tried not to let it show
Another strategy which Dan adopted under stress was to try not to let it show so that other members of staff did not start to panic. He became accustomed to the uncertainty of the working environment and did not think about it.

Kept up appearances
Much was expected of Ruth, who had to put on an act when she felt in a bad mood. Some days she felt it was really difficult to keep up an 'air hostess' façade over the things that were niggling her. She could not be herself because it was not what the patients expected – they were too busy being ill to be interested in her life, and she had to give the patients what they wanted.

❑ Theme 6: Superficial preparation for the job

Nearly all nurses commented on their training and professional preparation for the work. A distinct theme to emerge was the belief that people could be trained to carry out nursing procedures but not any form of emotional caring response.

Received a procedural training devoid of emotional content
Jeff was trained to care for people essentially through physical care skills, although he had also received some training in interpersonal and social skills, which helped his ability to care to develop. A number of the nurses interviewed believed that it was not possible to train people to care in any emotional sense; it was difficult to train people in the feeling side of caring.

It was felt that training showed people what was expected of them and helped them to achieve self-control and keep their views to themselves. It equipped nurses with the knowledge to answer patients' questions and give basic care, prepared nurses to cope with emergencies but did not really prepare them for the emotional facets of their role.

Needed training in physical and psychological care

Emma believed that physical and psychological care were different but that it was important to teach nurses to treat all people as individuals worthy of care. Not everyone agreed, however. Cath did not see any relationship between caring and professional nursing, although caring greatly influenced her professional conduct as a nurse. Similarly, Mona described professional caring as being able to do everything for the patient and act appropriately as the patient's condition changed. Both physical and psychological care were seen as part of caring for patients, and training in both aspects was felt to be needed.

Needed an intrinsic capacity to care

The training which most of the nurses received emphasised the procedural aspects of caring for patients. This was counterbalanced by a belief held by most of the nurses interviewed here that good carers had an intrinsic capacity to care. Jeff had this capacity as part of his make-up; he believed that nurses needed this intrinsic capacity to care for others but felt that not everyone had it. Emma also felt that caring was partly intrinsic; she was not conscious of having been taught to care. Trudy believed that people had to want to care, it had to be part of them:

> I don't know, it's just something they enjoy doing, they want to do. It's part of their personality. That's what they enjoy doing, that's what they want to do.

❏   Theme 7: Constrained by the ward environment

A number of nurses were of the view that the environment designed for nursing patients was sometimes unsuitable for that purpose and constrained the nurses' capacity to care for their patients.

Unsuitable ward environment

It was felt not to be good to have a psychiatric ward in a general hospital because of the difficulties of observation. Steve had to provide a therapeutic environment, although the setting for the ward was totally wrong and prevented him from doing so. The ward was a daunting place for some of the others, although Trish described the same ward as being well set up and busy.

Much time wasted on paperwork
As a staff nurse, Steve wasted much of his time on paperwork which was only remotely related to caring, although it was an important form of indirect care and someone had to do it properly. Paperwork could also be used to 'look busy' and shy away from clinical work. However, Steve felt that doing the paperwork was not right and that the emphasis in his work was wrongly placed.

Limited resources
The short supply of simple things such as flannels and soap on some wards restricted what could be done for patients, and there was felt to be a lack of private space for patients throughout the hospital.

Authoritarian consultant was dominant
It was difficult for Ruth and other nurses on a busy ward with an authoritarian consultant who usually gave out orders once a week and then disappeared.

The influential role of the ward sister
Ruth believed that the ward sisters had a crucial role to play in providing care for patients and promoting developments and changes in practice at ward level. A 'good' sister could make things happen while a 'poor' sister could limit other people.

Wasted time walking up and down the ward
Ruth believed she wasted much of her time walking up and down wards to get things because the layout of the ward was poor and inappropriate. The workload, the available time, and the atmosphere on the ward also affected her ability to care for patients.

Tried to ensure other staff kept the standards up
As a staff nurse, Ruth was responsible for maintaining good standards of care on the ward. She had to keep an eye on other staff to make sure that standards were appropriate, and she felt responsible for the quality of nursing care.

Limited time
Time also assumed great importance in caring for patients because it determined the quality of care given and the ability of staff to implement new ideas. Steve found that it was difficult to find the time to follow initiatives through from start to finish, the general lack of staff being only part of the problem. Mona also found it stressful when the ward was busy and there was no time to finish anything properly.

Personal limitations

Aine noted how her planned holiday interrupted her relationships with some patients, although she knew that this was inevitable from time to time. Others felt that their lack of professional expertise in some areas, such as coping with bereaved relatives, was a major limitation. When Ruth felt ill or had a bad day, she believed that she did not work well.

Good wards were less constraining

In contrast, some of the nurses worked on good wards. Jeff found himself working on a demanding ward which was also caring, and this helped him in his dealings with patients because he had supportive colleagues.

Good rapport between doctors and nurses

There was a clear division of responsibility between the doctors and the nurses, which helped to build up a good rapport between the different groups of professional staff. Dan worked on a ward where there was a good relationship between the doctors and the nurses; this helped to build up a team spirit, even when things got really busy.

❏ Theme 8: Coped with a demanding and uncertain role

Nearly all of the nurses engaged in some form of appraisal of their role as professional carers. They had to cope with the inherent demands which the role placed on them.

Doubts about being a nurse

Steve was still not sure that he really wanted to be a nurse – he did not see himself as a caring person. He sometimes asked himself: 'why am I here?' Ruth also felt that she had to decide on her role.

Experience promoted self-confidence

Although Emma had more time for patients as a student, she lacked confidence, but as a staff nurse she was more self-confident and her role was more fulfilling. She felt she had more information to give people and others were less likely to question her professionalism. Her experience helped her to give better care and assess patient needs, and people expected more of her now that she wore a blue uniform.

Freedom to care

Trish thought that her role as a nursing assistant gave her the freedom to care and do what she felt was appropriate for patients.

Wanted to help others

Trish wanted to help all patients; she could not stop herself being a carer even if she did not like a patient. She soon realised that this job was the job she really wanted to do.

Role ambiguity

A number of the nurses experienced a sense of ambiguity within their roles. Steve found it difficult to define the role of the mental health nurse; he was confused about what the staff nurse should be doing. Cath found that aspects of her role as a student prevented her from caring for patients in the way she wanted. Because she was inexperienced, she had to admit to patients when she did not know something, which conveyed a lot to patients and altered her relationship with them.

As a nursing assistant, Trudy found that her restricted training limited her ability to care. She did not tackle situations of which she was unsure but referred them on to some of the trained staff. Sometimes she had to ask permission to do certain things with patients, and she was unable to answer questions. The rules and regulations which had to be followed in some instances prevented her from caring for patients as she wanted to. Another nursing assistant, Trish, felt she was sometimes asked to do unimportant or stupid things by the qualified staff when that time could have been better spent with patients.

Role conflict

The qualified staff nurses found that the manager-carer role which they were expected to fill was a source of conflict, too many different demands within the role preventing things from being followed through. Steve found it difficult to decide what was more important from one day to the next. Emma also found the manager-carer conflict hard to resolve. As a staff nurse, Ruth felt that the emphasis was on management rather than care – even though patients were her first priority. Dan's role as a staff nurse prevented him from caring for patients as he wanted to because his time was taken up with administration. There was generally a greater emphasis on management within the staff nurse role, while students and enrolled nurses did more with patients. Dan missed the intimate contact with patients.

Management got in the way of patient care

Emma found that the managerial aspects of her role as a staff nurse stopped her from looking after patients and caused frequent interruptions when she was with patients and relatives. Aine's time for patients was limited by being in charge of the ward, as she had to concentrate on the risky psychotic patients. Just being with the patients caused Ruth difficulties in her staff nurse role because she was unable to give physical care and time to patients. Mona, on the other hand, was a state enrolled nurse, who was not bogged down by management tasks as were those nurses who took charge of the ward. She felt she was able to give basic care and develop technical skills such as giving intravenous drugs.

Pressure to conform
As a new staff nurse, Emma was under a lot of pressure to conform to her colleagues' and managers' traditional view of the staff nurse. Other staff expected her to meet their needs before those of the patient.

Patients did not bother the qualified staff
It was believed that patients perceived the qualified staff and doctors as being too busy for them. Aine thought that patients felt that the staff had no time for them, so they did not bother them but talked to the students and nursing assistants instead.

❏   Theme 9: Personal benefits derived from caring for others

The nurses derived much positive benefit from caring for patients despite the stresses and strains involved in the work.

Patient responded positively
Emma's patient recognised her interest and concern, and could distinguish caring nurses by the way they did simple things such as the routine observations of temperature, pulse and blood pressure. Cath's patient responded positively to her efforts – he smiled and was generally appreciative. Cath enjoyed being with him and even asked to be assigned to him when the senior staff were working out how staff should be allocated. Mona's support was gratefully appreciated by her patient, as she had helped to relieve the patient's loneliness.

Got through to the patient
Ruth gradually got to know her depressed patient, was able to get through to her when other staff could not, and tried to involve her even when she was unresponsive. When she talked to the patient, she expected a response, and she sometimes got one.

Positive contribution was gratifying
Making a positive contribution was rewarding for Steve, although positive results did not always follow his efforts. He got a sense of satisfaction because he was happy with his professional contribution, although from time to time he expected positive results to boost his own self-esteem. Cath felt really good to see people get better and go home.

Seeing patients as friends
Steve got a lot of satisfaction from seeing patients as ordinary people and friends with whom he shared things, but it was not always possible to do this. Occasionally, Steve went drinking with patients, which was not professional, but it sometimes got positive results. He felt that it was important to be able to get patients to accept care.

Being appreciated by patients
Patients were grateful to Emma and she enjoyed that feeling. Cath felt good that the patients wanted to talk to her and obviously needed her attention; talking to patients helped to motivate her. Trish was happy to be appreciated by the patients even though it was her job. She felt, however, that some patients saw her as a jailer, and she did not like the way they looked at her.

Doing something worthwhile
Trish liked working with people and liked the feeling of caring because she helped the patients to get well. Mona enjoyed surgical nursing and the quick turnover; she felt as though she was really doing something for very sick people. Dan needed to do something worthwhile and satisfying, and his job allowed him to do it.

Enjoyed the sense of achievement
The sense of achievement which caring for others provided was recognised by several nurses. Sometimes the patient responded; this gave Trudy a great sense of achievement at work. She enjoyed achieving things with patients, especially establishing and building a trusting relationship with them. Ruth enjoyed meeting people and was happy in her job; she was just pleased to be able to help somebody. Dan felt good when he achieved what he set out to do for patients and left the patients in a comfortable condition when he went home from work.

Learned a lot about people
Jeff learned a lot about people's problems and how they coped with them through caring for others. So, too, did Cath. Trudy found looking after and getting to know people interesting and enjoyable. She got along with most people and learned a great deal from patients which helped her to be aware of her own reactions to situations outside work. Aine also felt that she learned a lot about personal relationships in her work.

Personal development
Ruth benefited by developing and changing personally. She grew up quickly and it brought out qualities which would not otherwise have emerged: she became responsible, respected and trusted. Emma benefited

by having the opportunity to look at her own feelings and reactions to situations and people. Mona learned how families coped with death, and she became less frightened. She learned how to reassure bereaved families and used this skill outside the hospital. Emma found that caring increased her self-worth, giving her a sense of being trustworthy and of being trusted.

■ Summary

The findings provide a very rich and detailed analysis of what it means to care for patients in a professional nursing context. The social context of the ward environment – busy surgical wards, quiet medical wards, acute psychiatric admission – all influence the way nurses care for patients – limiting or enhancing their responses. The nurses were constantly aware of the stresses and constraints imposed by the system. The level of involvement with patients was influenced by the nurses' need to be able to achieve positive feedback for their efforts on the one hand and avoid the risks and stresses entailed in over-involvement with patients and work on the other.

The next chapter examines the views and experiences of patients.

■ Further reading

Koch, T. 1995 Interpretive approaches in nursing research: the influence of Husserl and Heidegger. *Journal of Advanced Nursing*, **21**(5):827–36.

Koch, T., Webb, C. and Williams, A.M. 1995 Listening to the voices of older patients: an existential–phenomenological approach to quality assurance. *Journal of Clinical Nursing*, **4**(3):185–93.

Larson-Presswalla, J., Rose, M.A. and Cornett, P. 1995 Empathic learning: an innovative teaching strategy to improve attitudes toward caring for persons with HIV/AIDS. *Journal of the Association of Nurses in AIDS Care*, **6**(3):19–22.

Chapter Five

Being cared for

Nurses need to *understand* what it feels like to be a patient in order to be able to care. In this chapter, we describe some patients' experiences of 'being cared for' in hospital. The portrait of the patients' experiences highlights the need for quality psychological care in the hospital environment. As in the previous chapter, the methodological details are omitted; those interested in finding out more should read Morrison (1991, 1992).

■ The interviews with patients

The approach used to study patients' experiences was informed by existential phenomenology – the primary aim being to study human experience from the point of view of the person being studied (Taylor and Bogdan, 1984). This approach has become very popular in health care and nursing research. It has been claimed that phenomenologically based health care research provides a powerful set of techniques for exploring patient and professional viewpoints (Kestenbaum, 1982a). Moreover, Kestenbaum (1982a) suggested that these different perspectives could help to re-shape professional practice and policies.

A purposive sample of 10 patients (informants) from medical and surgical wards were asked to talk about their experiences of 'being cared for'. These patients were selected in discussions with the senior nursing staff on the wards. The interviews were guided by a small set of questions that focused on *what* the nurses did for patients and *how* they did their work. The patients were ordinary people who were willing, and well enough, to talk freely about their experiences in hospital.

All the patients in the study were inpatients in a large teaching hospital and varied in age, diagnosis, prognosis, sex and length of time spent in hospital. Some were in hospital for the first time, while others had had a number of previous admissions to this or other hospitals. The interviews were tape-recorded and later transcribed word for word. This procedure produced a very detailed and rich picture of the patients' experiences. The remainder of this chapter outlines a summary of the main findings.

■ The main themes in the patient interviews

Four major themes characterised the patients' accounts of being cared for. These were:

1. patients experienced crushing vulnerability
2. patients adopted a particular mode of self-presentation
3. patients evaluated the hospital services, and
4. patients' personal concerns assumed great importance.

These themes form the remainder of this chapter. Limitations of space mean that only the main findings will be discussed; some of these will include direct quotations from the patients themselves. Under each of the main themes, a number of sub-themes are described. These illustrate many different aspects of the experience of the main themes. The themes and sub-themes are organised and laid out like those in the previous chapter.

❏ Theme 1: Patients experienced crushing vulnerability

Patients experienced being cared for as a time of crushing vulnerability. The uncertainty associated with being ill and in hospital was a particularly powerful emotional response.

The hospital environment was strange
The hospital was a intimidating place for a number of patients and evoked feelings of intense vulnerability and uncertainty about what they should do in this strange place. James, a 67-year-old retired headmaster, stated:

> I don't like being in a situation that I don't know what to do.

Zoe was frightened and felt she now had no control over her situation, having to rely fully on the staff. It was felt that patients were in hospital because they *had* to be there – James was there under duress.

While patients were uncertain and very vulnerable, some patients found that they were better able to cope with the hospital environment, especially those who had been patients before or who were spending a long time in hospital. This was not always true, however – one patient, Martha, had spent several weeks in hospital after extensive plastic surgery.

Although she knew the staff well and felt well cared for, she found herself crying from time to time because being in hospital just 'got to her'.

Anxiety about being treated like an object

The approach which staff employ when interacting with patients can lead to anxiety. Several patients found that being in hospital induced anxiety over being *treated like an object*. For example, James did not want to become just a name on a sheet of paper. Unfortunately, this feeling can all too easily be created by staff in any hospital as they interact *routinely* with patients. Many nurses and doctors regularly refer to people in hospital as 'patients', 'schizophrenics', 'diabetics', and so on, and this can all too easily degenerate into the type of non-person treatment that patients experience.

Hugh's feelings were completely ignored by staff. He found that he, too, was completely ignored during the handovers which were often carried out at the foot of Hugh's bed as if he did not exist. The lack of privacy was also felt to be embarrassing. Hugh wanted the nurses to talk *to* him but instead the staff talked *about* him as if he did not exist:

> it's almost as if you're being talked about and are not there. You know, this is Mr D. who had a bath… *I'm here…*

Positive impact of being treated like a person

Some patients commented on the positive impact of being 'treated like a person', which made them feel better and boosted their confidence. Others felt that being treated like a person promoted recovery and had a positive effect on their health. Although the staff did nothing dramatic for Florence, they just made her:

> feel like a person, you know, not a number…

which helped her to relax and get better. Some patients liked the staff to call them by their first name, but not all did. For some, it appears to promote positive feelings, but for others it may promote unease and be interpreted as a lack of respect.

The nursing staff were friendly and did not make Florence feel 'small'. Eileen was sure that the nurses would always respect her wishes and would not take advantage of her. Another patient, Tim, had a very positive experience when he returned to the ward after being sent to another hospital for a series of diagnostic investigations:

> When they seen me come back here last week young Jane got hold of me as if she hadn't seen me for donkeys years, as if I was a long lost brother or something. They made me feel like somebody…

Shattering impact of cancer

Some of the patients faced a poor prognosis. Two had recently been diagnosed as having cancer, which had had a tremendous impact on their lives and on their families. Both patients who developed cancer 'needed to know the truth' about their condition and 'the future'. None of the doctors would tell Tim 'the worst' directly, which made him feel even more anxious. When he was finally learned the truth, he was very hurt because the doctor and his wife had 'conspired' to keep him in the dark.

When Tim 'discovered' he had lung cancer he went numb and then went to pieces. Gradually, he came to accept his diagnosis. Al's experience of cancer differed. In the beginning, it all seemed like nothing to him – a small mole on his back which was eventually diagnosed as skin cancer. The professor told him that he had cancer, that it was very serious and that the prognosis was not good.

Not surprisingly, these patients spent time 'thinking about dying and death'. When Al found out he had terminal cancer, he found himself in hospital thinking about his life:

> life is sweet. I've got a little car, a wife and two nice children and we go and do things. Not a lot of money but it's nice. You know... after working all your life and retiring now comes the sallow days.

Patients wanted to have 'hope'. During his first operation, Al had a melanoma removed. The operation went well, but he knew that there were 'no guarantees' even though everything that could be done surgically had been done. Some time after the first operation, another lump was discovered at an outpatient appointment, and a second operation was needed. This went well, too. All Al felt he could do now was to wait and see.

Traumatic investigations and surgery

Tim had to undergo a period of lengthy and drawn-out investigations, which he found very traumatic.

Cancelled operation was a major setback

A cancelled operation led Tim to assume that the cancer had spread to other parts of his body. He calmed down after hearing that the operation was not cancelled completely but rather postponed until all his test results were available.

Anxious suspicion

Tim felt that if the nurses pampered him or spent too much time with him, he would have suspected that something was seriously wrong:

If they kept on I'm sure I'd think there was more wrong than is actually the case. That's how I would feel if they pampered me too much. I'd know. That I do believe.

Surrendering independence was distressing
Martha's lengthy stay in hospital was necessary because she needed a series of skin graft operations. She had to give up her independence, felt clumsy at having to be helped to the toilet and was very distressed:

> I found it very difficult, very upsetting. I really thought that after six weeks I was going back to stage one.

Martha regained her independence gradually as the staff withdrew their help in a systematic manner.

Coping with bodily disfigurement was traumatic
Martha found her skin graft very unpleasant to look at, and at first she felt like 'fainting'. Eventually, she had to accept that she had a stoma and reached a point where she looked after herself independently.

Difficult being away from home for a long time
Martha was unexpectedly away from home and relatives for more than 8 weeks and her family could only visit her at weekends. She felt that staff should have spent more time with her but that they were 'overly professional' and distant.

Felt like a smelly mess compared with the nurses
Zoe messed the floor because she had diarrhoea and felt 'awful' because the student nurse had to clean it up. When she compared herself with the nurses, who were well groomed, she said she felt like a 'smelly mess'.

Felt forgotten about
There was one occasion when Ed felt forgotten about, having to wait for over 5 hours for the doctor to come and set up an intravenous drip. Although Ed felt neglected by the staff, he still defended them by emphasising how busy the nurses and doctors were:

> as I was saying there were other things doing and all. I don't suppose they can be in two places at once. But you're not the only one, I expect there were others worse than I was like, that needed attending to.

COMMENT

Being ill and admitted to hospital is very anxiety provoking, a feeling probably shared by most patients and their families. The whole process contributes to feelings of 'crushing vulnerability' and offers opportunities for providing good psychological care. 'Crushing vulnerability' emphasises each patient's need for sensitive nursing care.

Only one patient of the 10 interviewed here was openly critical of the general care he received, because he was made to feel like an 'object'. He reported that he had little say in his overall management, he was ignored during handovers, his personal details were discussed publicly by staff and he had little contact with the trained staff. All these subtle, and not so subtle, actions made him feel like an 'object'.

❏   **Theme 2: Patients adopted a particular mode of self-presentation**

Several patients noted changes in their own behaviour that were linked to being ill and in hospital. They adopted particular modes of self-presentation, in some cases consciously and in others without awareness. Below are given some of the modes of presentation that were identified during the analysis of the interviews.

Became sheepishly obedient
Some patients became very obedient. Florence for example, did everything that the staff told her to do:

Maybe I'm a bit sheepish.

She looked to the doctors, nurses and other professionals when things went wrong because she had 'blind faith' in them. James, too, was led by the needs of the staff and made sure that he always gave staff the 'correct information'. He did not want to waste time because they were busy, and he did what was asked of him unquestioningly.

Although Tim was very anxious, he had to be examined by lots of medical students because of his 'complicated and medically interesting' condition. He put up with all the examinations and probing because he did not want to look foolish by not co-operating with those who were treating him.

Conformed to the ritualistic practice

Other patients found themselves conforming to ritualistic routines. George was not 'allowed' to collect his medicine from the medicine trolley, although he collected his own tea from the tea trolley.

Became unusually friendly and cheerful

Some patients coped with the anxieties and uncertainties that the hospital aroused in different ways. One strategy, which is warmly welcomed by the staff, is to adopt an unusually friendly and cheerful disposition. Several patients adopted a cheerfulness that was unfitting for the awful situations in which they found themselves as they felt 'obliged' to try to be cheerful.

Provided a frank and honest account

One patient displayed an attitude of openness and honesty, which meant that the staff learned a great deal about him and his life while he knew nothing about them. This is a routine practice and the 'accepted' way to proceed in a hospital context. Through this imbalance, the patient's vulnerability is heightened while the power and status of the professional carer may be enhanced.

George told the truth about his excessive drinking as not to tell the whole truth could damage his chances of recovery through inappropriate treatment. However, disclosing information about his drinking exposed him to the risk of being sanctioned or ignored by the staff like an unpopular patient because conditions associated with 'drinking' may be attributed to being the patient's own fault.

Helpful camaraderie amongst patients

Patients of different backgrounds and cultures are often thrown together by chance through the experience of illness. They are drawn closer together both physically and psychologically because staff and relatives spend so little time with them. Patients often develop a comradeship between themselves to support each other; they make a point of helping each other.

The enforced camaraderie in the hospital ward helps to reduce boredom and pass the time as much of the patients' day is spent 'waiting'. These small groups are also likely to help patients to talk about their illness, investigations, treatments, and so on as a way of dealing with anxiety, although some patients may find these informal conversations anxiety provoking.

Reluctant to ask questions

In this setting, patients were not encouraged to question the staff, and this may be a characteristic of life in hospital. When patients did ask questions, the staff appeared to employ subtle tactics for letting the patients know that they should not – letting the patient know how busy they were, giving the impression that the patient was being a nuisance, or providing incomplete answers to the patient's questions. These tactics had the effect of closing down any further communication.

Several patients wanted and needed more information. Some refrained from asking questions altogether, while others limited their questioning to questions begging a simple 'yes' or 'no' answer. This meant that the questions did not make the staff feel uneasy and lead to upsetting situations. Most patients were acutely aware of their lack of knowledge of what was going on around them.

One way of ensuring that patients did not ask searching questions was to give the impression of 'business'. There is, in the hospital culture, a tacit obligation to 'look busy', and this was obviously noted by some patients. The patients in this study were not encouraged to ask questions, although James said nobody had actually told him *not to*. Hugh was made to feel like a nuisance for asking questions, especially of the doctors.

Kept interpersonal encounters superficial

A number of patients kept their interactions with others brief and superficial. James limited his interactions with others in the ward and did not say a lot about his illness, talking instead about such superficial things as the weather, sport and the television. Close relationships with nurses were not considered:

> It's me. That's the way I am, that's the way I've lived. I'm an ex-headmaster, I've had to learn to draw lines.

George kept to himself and read, whereas Ed felt that the nurses did what they had to do and no more – nurses were not interested in, nor supposed to get closer to, patients in hospital.

Tried not to be a nuisance

A number of patients tried not to be a 'nuisance'. James kept out of the way, especially when the staff were ill-tempered:

> they come on to a shift at seven in the morning after getting up at six
> and people can get up out of the wrong side of the bed. If you notice
> that, you know to keep your head down.

Martha suggested that 'not being a nuisance' meant that other patients got their fair share of care and attention from the staff, but she was sometimes made to feel *guilty* by the staff, who let her know that other patients on the ward needed caring for too.

Provided a sense of purpose for the carers
Although in a very vulnerable position, some patients felt that they were able to give something back to the staff who cared for them, such as a sense of achievement.

Showed deference and gratitude to the carers
Patients were generally very grateful for the care they received from the staff. Al always displayed good manners and 'thanks' to the people who looked after him; he really appreciated what was done for him and treated the staff respectfully.

Admired the hard-working staff
There was much admiration for the work done by the 'dedicated' staff for the patients in their care. Zoe could not understand how the nurses did some of the 'awful jobs' which they had to do.

COMMENT

The patients adopted different roles while in hospital. They needed to be seen by the staff as people 'worthy' of care by being vulnerable and in need of help. They also had to maintain their self-esteem.

A number of strategies of self-presentation were used. Some patients became very obedient and conformed to the ritualistic practices of the ward. However, this type of compliance may be dangerous (Ley, 1988). Other patients became unusually cheerful and friendly in a situation that was terrifying and anxiety provoking for them and probably also for their relatives. These strategies of self-presentation are likely to be well received by the staff and fit in well within the organisational culture. Cheerful, deferential and compliant patients are much more 'popular' than articulate, awkward and questioning patients (Stockwell, 1972). In another research study, Waterworth and Luker (1990) emphasised the importance of 'toeing the line' as a patient. Showing admiration for the dedicated staff ensured that patients would be seen in a positive light. These self-presentation 'tactics' helped patients to cope with anxiety.

❑   Theme 3: Patients evaluated the hospital services

Most patients evaluate the care they receive and the environment where care is given. In this study, patients were generally positive about their care and treatment, but there were examples of patients who were critical of the staff and the hierarchical organisation.

General level of satisfaction with the caring staff

Patients, as consumers, were generally very satisfied with the care they received and were genuinely indebted for what was done for them. The technical facets of the nurses' role were prominent in their evaluations. In addition Ed felt that hospital was the best place for him because there was nobody to look after him at home, and Florence just knew that the staff were 'doing their best' for her.

The level of contact between the professional carers and the patients was very limited. Some patients had a lot of direct nursing care but others did not have any 'real' nursing (basic/physical nursing care), only 'tests' such as chest X-rays and blood and urinary investigations. These 'self-caring' patients secured a very limited amount of nursing time. However, some of the patients felt that 'staff let the patients know they were there for them if they really needed them'.

Contact with the nurses was limited to the times when they had to perform routine tasks that were completed hastily. The limited contact between the nurses and some of the patients could mean that the psychological care of patients was lacking in this context. However, it is also important to note that basic or physical care presents the nurse with an opportunity for 'talking' to the patients, listening carefully to their point of view and assessing them psychologically.

Other patients needed a great deal of physical care. Zoe had to be helped in and out of the bath initially and then helped to walk until she regained her independence. The nursing staff tried to thwart any tendency for Zoe to become over-dependent.

Staff were friendly but diplomatic

Although the contact between patients and nursing staff was limited, several patients commented on the positive effect of having 'friendly' nursing staff around. Although the staff were friendly, Zoe noted that they were also 'careful' and 'diplomatic' when talking about her illness.

Nurses asked what the patients needed

Because Martha was confined to bed for a long time without frequent visitors, some of the nurses made a point of asking if she needed washing or shopping done. One young student nurse took Martha's dressing gown home overnight and washed it; others brought in magazines for her to look at to help pass the time and lessen the boredom.

Felt safe and trusted the nurses

The nurses had to do a lot for Martha, and she trusted the nurses and felt at ease with them. They held her firmly when she had to get into the bath, although she said that some nurses made her feel safer than others.

Technical competence was appreciated

Patients were full of praise for the nursing skill and expertise – injections were administered competently and sensitively, medicines were given on time, blood samples were taken quickly and proficiently, and the experienced nurses were good at dealing with drips and dressings. The nurses made constant checks on the patients and responded promptly when someone rang a call bell. They were perceived by the patients to be 'always on their toes'.

The approach of the staff was sensitive and calming

The nurses' ability to calm Tim without minor tranquilizers when he was very anxious was important. When Al came into hospital, he had been very apprehensive, but he felt that the staff had quickly dispelled his fears. George watched the nurses and doctors in action from a distance. He overheard things as the nurses calmed a very frightened patient by just sitting him down and arranging for a social worker to help his lonely disabled wife.

When Martha's husband came to visit her at the weekend, the nurses gave her husband a spare meal so that he could stay with her and avoid having to go down to the canteen some distance from the ward. The staff knew he had travelled a long distance to be with her and in a few short hours would have to go home again to look after Martha's sick mother. This 'bending of the rules' showed Martha that the nursing staff really understood her loneliness.

The accommodation and hotel services were reasonable

Accommodation and hotel services also emerged as an important issue in patients' evaluations of hospital. In general, the quality of the food was good and the bed linen was changed daily. However, one of the patients noted that the china was cracked and ought to have been replaced. Zoe found the hospital to be clean and tidy.

The devoted students were constantly available

The student nurses were singled out by several patients for their attentive care and devotion, the younger nurses always being available. The patients did not object to the fact that they were looked after mainly by student nurses rather than trained and experienced nurses, because these young nurses had to get experience to fulfil their training requirements. The 'constant availability' of the students was very notable and much appreciated.

The students spent more time with the patients and got to know them better than the qualified staff did. The students took time to talk to patients and shared 'a bit of their lives'. They were good listeners and often stayed on late to finish their work. Not all the patients, however, were particularly appreciative of the students' approach. Ed had little contact with students and noted how the students just went around with the doctors. In general, the staff tended to ignore him.

Helped to get through the miserable nights

The nights were mentioned by several patients as being difficult. It was a time that Zoe found particularly hard because she could not sleep well. She found herself tired but restless at night, and felt it was unpleasant to be woken up so early in the morning to fit in with the ward routine. Some patients found the night staff very helpful because they made tea during the night to help patients sleep – just as would happen at home. The night staff told Zoe how well her wound was healing, and they reassured her about her progress.

Did not get to know nurses well

It is often claimed that the relationship between patients and nurses is the foundation for providing good nursing care. It was notable that patients did not get to know any of the nurses, and contact between patients and nurses was often limited to 'tablet time'. Nevertheless, some patients did not see a need to get to know the nurses well: they just wanted to be looked after by competent staff who treated them like 'people'.

The trained nurses, unlike the students, spent even less time interacting with the patients. Hugh, for example, did not even speak to the ward sister at any time during his stay in hospital. The lack of contact with trained staff made a big difference to the patients' day. One of them commented how the qualified staff *found things for the students to do* if they saw them talking to patients or sitting down at the patients' bedsides.

The contact between trained nursing staff and patients tended to be rather superficial. George just passed the time of day with staff by talking about the weather, the television, the most recent news items, and so on. Some interactions with patients were limited to the nurse asking a patient to get off his bed so that it could be made up.

In addition, the patients generally perceived the staff as being 'too busy' to talk to them, or felt that other more serious patients needed attention urgently. Several patients commented that the nurses were too busy and did not have time to talk:

> The nurses didn't talk about the operation because they're awfully busy, they'll talk to you – yes. 'How are you today? How's your wound? Lets have a look at it, that's fine that's coming on nicely'. That sort of thing. But I mean they are awfully busy and there is a lot of physical work attached…

It was suggested that the really ill patients needed lots of attention and rest and that the staff had to get on with their difficult work. One patient felt that some staff *gave the impression* of being understaffed, while others were always relaxed and ensured that patients were well cared for no matter what pressure they were under.

Nothing was too much trouble

The attitude of the caring nurses was captured by several patients in this sub-theme. Zoe felt that the staff were genuinely busy but still gave the impression that 'nothing was too much trouble'. They got the phone for her on many occasions and placed it beside her bed so that she could phone home. Paying attention to small details can make a big difference to the quality of care that patients experience.

No front – just genuine nurses

Tim felt that there was no 'front' to the nurses' attitude: they always displayed a concern 'for his well-being' and it was a genuine concern. Hugh described the approach of the students as genuine and not patronising – the qualified nurses he felt were, however, different.

Displayed a caring attitude in their work

The nurses had time for the 'personal touch' that was important for George – he described this as a 'caring attitude' and it showed in the way they looked after the patients on the ward.

The doctors were approachable

Some doctors too were singled out for comment because they were 'good and introduced themselves' to the patients when they came to the bedside. This made them more human and less frightening. The doctors allowed Florence to ask questions, and she felt more confident when she did. Another patient felt that the doctors were 'exceptional'.

Key criticisms of the staff

Several important criticisms of the staff also emerged; these highlighted the need for staff to listen carefully to what patients have to say. The importance of good manners was highlighted. George commented on the rude tea ladies, one of whom 'almost threw the tea' at him, and on the auxiliary nurse who was particularly rude. Zoe had an upsetting argument with a rude receptionist about her special diet, becoming very upset and very angry about the whole incident, which could easily have been avoided.

Hurried approach of the nurses provoked anxiety

Martha did not like it when the nurses were 'in a rush' – especially when she was in pain. Being rushed made her feel 'on edge', and the nurses tended to 'dash through their work' when they were short of staff. Zoe needed regular baths and noticed that the busy auxiliaries were constantly trying to get her into the bath in a rather 'hurried' fashion.

Kept in the dark
Some patients were not given enough information about their illness, treatment and what would happen to them. There was a general lack of information on some wards; some patients even had to ask what their tablets were for, which most wanted to know. Several patients were not told why certain things were done and this seemed like the routine:

> there's a definite lack of information. They do things but you don't know why half of the time.

It was even suggested that the staff were 'trained to keep people in the dark'.

Boredom
One of the biggest problems in hospitals is boredom. Hospital became boring for Zoe and there were no organised activities on the ward, so she was left to 'entertain' herself by whatever means she could during the day. This situation meant that most patients were left to 'wait' and think about what might happen to them.

COMMENT

Many positive comments on the nurses' performance emerged – the friendliness, their concerns for patients and their technical competence were all greatly appreciated by patients. The fact that any criticisms came out is surprising because of the vulnerability of this patient group. Patients focused on things that may seem trivial and routine to the staff. However, it has been suggested that suggested that the routine 'services' greatly influence patients' perceptions of care and the expressed level of satisfaction with services (Rempusheski *et al.*, 1988). Having clean bed linen, or a clean and uncracked cup to drink out of, has symbolic meaning for patients, conveying a message that the patient is a *person worthy of care*, and not an object.

The student nurses and the night staff were singled out for praise, but qualified and more senior nursing staff may need to think carefully about their role. Are they providers of direct patient care or managers of such services? The trained staff were generally perceived by patients as being too busy for them. This finding supports the general tendency for much of the basic nursing to be done in particular by the learners or by untrained staff (Knight and Field, 1981; Robinson *et al.*, 1989).

It is important to note that patients are usually very reluctant to voice any criticism of the staff to anyone remotely involved in the system. This may be the result of an implicit rule of being a vulnerable patient – never criticise – because criticism is likely to lead to patients being labelled 'good' or 'bad' (Lorber, 1975; Kelly and May, 1982) or unpopular (Stockwell, 1972) and treated accordingly. Most of the official complaints about hospital highlight 'poor communication' as the major source of patient dissatisfaction (Audit Commission, 1993).

Ask yourself how well you deal with patient complaints. Discuss this with some colleagues and listen to their views. Consider reviewing the channels of communication that exist in places where you have worked. Identify 'good' and 'poor' communication practices in those places. Do you continue to apply the good principles?

❏ Theme 4: Patients' personal concerns assumed great importance

It was apparent that the patients' personal concerns were not always recognised by the staff. The personal concerns of patients may influence their perceptions of the context in which care is experienced. The personal concerns mentioned here cannot reflect the concerns of *all* patients but give instead a small flavour of what may be an important source of patient anxiety but go unnoticed by staff.

The treatment was primary
The *treatment* was the most important aspect of being in hospital. Patients may perceive the nurse's role as primarily one of ensuring that patients get the right treatment. This was certainly the case with James, who was concerned only about his treatment – nothing else mattered to him. Ed likewise just needed an operation to put things right; then he could get out of the hospital and resume his normal life outside.

Nurses can also make an effort to improve the quality of *that individual's care* by being well informed about his or her treatment and medical management and ensuring that patients are kept up to date. The importance of the nurse's role in giving information to patients and their relatives has been widely demonstrated (see for example Devine and Cook, 1983).

Being in hospital was frustrating
Hospitalisation can be a very frustrating time for patients. A person's whole life may be radically altered by illness: work, social life and personal relationships can be seriously disrupted. In some cases, such as life-threatening illness, unexpected trauma or the diagnosis of a stigmatising illness such as

'breast cancer' or 'schizophrenia', a person's life may be ruined. While some patients may be in hospital for investigations and are obviously not acutely 'ill', others may be there for life-saving surgery, to have children or for more long-term treatment.

Frustration can result from different sources, such as having to ask a nurse for a 'bottle'. Hugh was disheartened because he felt pretty well in himself but he *had to stay in bed* and use a commode beside the bed in a ward with other patients. Many patients in hospital are referred to as 'self-caring' during the daily report because they do not need much direct nursing, yet these individuals are often subject to the same restrictive regimes that many acutely ill patients willingly undergo without question. This was certainly the case with some of the patients interviewed in this study.

Felt let down by the GP after husband's death

During her interview Florence talked a lot about her GP, who was very supportive when her husband died. He was one of those doctors who was 'always available and willing to talk' to her about the death of her husband and her own health. Since her husband died, Florence too had become ill and needed to make more frequent calls on the GP service. As time went by, Florence began to feel 'neglected' and 'let down' by the GP and his colleagues, who lacked patience. Eventually, Florence saw the consultant surgeon, and this led to her admission to hospital for surgery.

Mother's recent death

During the interview, Eileen talked about how her mother had died just before she had to come into hospital. Eileen had to deal with the death, the funeral and its aftermath, and this experience was with her constantly as she found herself in hospital and in need of treatment. This is a particularly good example of the nurses' need to take account of the important events that may be happening or have recently happened to a person who arrives on the ward as a patient. Helping patients to deal with these personal experiences may, however, cause some conflict with colleagues who may have a more 'detached' approach to patients (Menzies, 1970).

The previous admission to hospital was terrible

Previous admissions to hospital can help the patient to come into hospital in a more settled state of mind or they can generate stifling anxiety. George described his previous admission to hospital for major surgery for a damaged kidney. It was a very traumatic experience for him because he was discharged before he had fully recovered, simply to free up beds for new patients.

Concerned about the family and close friends

The final topic to emerge as an important aspect of the patients' personal concerns dealt with their families and friends. At times of illness, people get physical and psychological support from other family members. Unfortunately, some patients lack support and may themselves be the major supportive force in the lives of others. This was the case for Martha and Ed.

Martha's mother, for example, lived over 250 miles away from the hospital, and she herself needed an operation to save the sight in her one good eye. She needed Martha to look after her, but Martha was stranded in hospital with no chance of a speedy recovery and discharge. Martha's mother and husband were all the family she had, and being far away from them was a 'constant source of worry'.

Ed was very concerned for the one 'visitor' who came to see him every day. She had to travel into the hospital by public transport, which meant she had to change buses twice, taking over an hour to get there. It was a long way for an elderly person, and the travelling took up much of her day. Ed was grateful that she came to see him, but he was 'worried about her health' because she had arthritis in her leg and was 'not very good on her feet'. She found it very difficult to get around and waiting for buses in bad weather was not good for her.

COMMENT

This theme emphasised more, very personal details of patients' experiences that may go unnoticed by staff. The personal concerns of the patients, however, serve as an important reminder of life outside hospital and the need for patients to continue to deal with external issues and relationships. Nurses need to set aside time to learn about these personal concerns. Staff may be able to offer support and, where appropriate, practical help.

Have you ever asked yourself what it must be like to use a commode? Do you actively talk to patients and family members to uncover potential sources of anxiety?

■ Summary

This detailed account of patients' experiences of being cared for in hospital emphasises the need for high-quality nursing care. The issues to emerge here will help you to think carefully about your own approach to patients and their families. An in-depth insight into patients' experiences is needed if nurses are to develop a sound *understanding* of patients and provide care that is both appropriate and effective. The rich and detailed findings that are described in this chapter illustrate how a phenomeno-logical approach may be used to enhance other approaches to the study of nurse–patient interactions.

■ Further reading

Beck, C.T. 1992 Caring among nursing students. *Nurse Educator*, **17**(6):22–7.
Bulmer, C.A. 1994 Maximum insight with minimum dependence: brief therapy in psychiatric nursing. *Professional Nurse*, **9**(9):621–5.
Crowden, A. 1994 On the moral nature of nursing practice. *Journal of Advanced Nursing*, **20**(6):1104–10.

PART TWO

Communicating and Nursing

Chapter Six

What is an interpersonally skilled nurse?

Caring is an *interpersonal* process, and the rapport between the carer and cared-for individual will be an important mediating force. It will influence the way in which the people perceive and interact with each other. Carers need interpersonal skills in order to get on with others and help them. The nature and scope of this interpersonal relationship needs also to be considered if we are to get a fuller understanding of how caring can be experienced. Successful interactions with others also form the basis of effective teamwork across professional boundaries in institutions and in the community.

In the next few chapters, we explore the notion of interpersonal and communication skills in nursing. We describe how a group of professional nurses defined the notion of an 'interpersonally skilled nurse'. It will be interesting to compare the findings of this study with those described in previous chapters. In nursing, is it *caring* that counts, or is it *being skilled*, or is it a mixture of both?

■ What is an interpersonal skill?

There are a number of models of interpersonal skill. However, a wide range of talents and abilities can actually be called interpersonal skills, a list of which would include some of the following: counselling, group membership skills, assertiveness, social skills, interviewing skills of various sorts, writing skills, using the telephone and group facilitation skills. Skills like these may be used when caring for others in some of the following ways:

- counselling skills: listening and talking to the distressed or depressed person

- assertiveness skills: coping with the 'difficult' client, working within a bureaucracy
- social skills: dealing with the general public, introductions to clients, visiting clients in their own homes, and
- facilitation skills: managing groups for educational purposes, facilitating therapy groups.

A lengthy and detailed discussion of the nature of interpersonal skills may be found elsewhere (Burnard, 1989a). Our intention here is to focus on *counselling skills* in nursing and explore counselling – as it relates to nursing – through a small qualitative study.

■ Counselling skills

Counselling skills may be used in a wide range of health care contexts. They may be used to help the person who is suffering from a temporary emotional crisis or in caring for the person who has longer-term problems in living. They may also be practical and useful as a set of interpersonal skills for everyday use in every client–practitioner situation. There is a considerable literature on counselling, and the reader is referred to this for further information about counselling theory and practice (Rogers, 1967; Burnard, 1994; Nelson-Jones, 1995). In this section, we report on a small-scale study that explored the notion of counselling in nursing.

■ A study of counselling in nursing

Although much has been written about counselling, there has – to date – been little research into counselling in nursing. In this qualitative and descriptive study, we sought the views of a small group of nurses who fulfilled either or both of the following criteria: (1) they were trained counsellors and nurses, and (2) they taught counselling skills to nurses.

Six nurses who fulfilled one or both of the above criteria were invited to take part in in-depth interviews with one of the writers. The interviews were transcribed and their content analysed into a series of themes. What follows is an elaboration of the findings accompanied by a commentary on the responses. The form of content analysis was that described by various qualitative researchers (Field and Morse, 1985; Miles and Huberman, 1994). The aim was to explore the data and to organise them according to emergent themes. These themes were partly dictated by the semi-structured interview schedule and partly by combing through the data and noting particular issues that were discussed by respondents. The aim was always to account for *all* of the data that arose out of the study.

Note how the methodological approach used in this chapter leads us to present the 'findings' in a particular way and how these are quite different from the findings reported in the previous two chapters.

❏ Counselling defined

Respondents offered various definitions of counselling. Sometimes those definitions referred to the *purpose* or *application* of counselling:

> I think that it is any kind of assistance in helping people to come to terms with an emotional or spiritual problem of any kind. It is not confined to mental distress or mental disorder. It can range from things like being in debt to having acute depression.

> Counselling is an activity in which one person is helping and one is receiving help and in which the emphasis of that help is on enabling the other person to find solutions to problems or to look at particular situations which they would like resolved. Or to enable them to live more resourcefully. It involves the development, by the counsellor, of a range of particular skills but more importantly the adoption of a particular stance or attitude towards the person being helped, and that includes the person feeling valued and able to explore the way in which he perceives himself and his world and not to feel judged by the counsellor.

> I think counselling is an activity in which two people agree to meet under certain conditions. And these conditions may be overt and negotiated and include such issues as confidentiality and expected outcomes. It is very much an interpersonal activity and the counsellor is there to help the client address and possibly resolve issues that are personal and meaningful to that individual.

One respondent referred to the need for the counsellor to remain *ordinary*. This idea of ordinariness in interpersonal relationships has been referred to elsewhere (Morrison, 1994). The argument is that people are likely to respond more readily to someone who does not attempt to assume a 'professional' front or one that is in any way 'artificial':

> For me, it is a means of just being with another person who may need to talk over problems, job difficulties, personal dilemmas and so forth. In much the same way as you talk things over with a spouse or friend. That *ordinariness*, if you like, is important in counselling.

Another respondent discussed counselling in terms of 'helping people to help' – a point that the respondent felt was echoed in the literature on the topic:

> Counselling is creating an environment in which people can explore the issues – whatever they are, whether it is a particular way of looking at life, a childhood issue, perhaps – in a supportive atmosphere. One official definition is helping people to help themselves and I quite like that: I think it's a good synopsis.

❑   The differences between counselling and psychotherapy

There has been some debate, in the literature, about what the differences between counselling and psychotherapy are. While, for some, psychotherapy is seen as 'deeper' and 'longer term', this is not always the case. The question was thus raised in this study as to what the difference between the two might be. Respondents reported as follows:

> Psychotherapy specifically applies to a clinical and mental illness as opposed to the run of the mill neuroses that run through society. Psychotherapy is done by psychotherapists (as opposed to counsellors) who can be lay therapists or qualified ones, whereas counselling can be done by a whole range of people, from priests to professional counsellors.

> I would guess that counselling would have a much more practical, every day, problem-solving slant to it – grounded in the here-and-now. Whereas psychotherapy, for me, evokes ideas to do with Freudian psychology, where a very specific type of framework might be used.

> I would see counselling as being more focused, more specific and more situationally oriented and I would see psychotherapy as much more a global view of the person's life, seeking to make changes which may affect the whole of the person's life, or seeking to make changes in a person's personality. I would see psychotherapy as exploring the person's life at a much deeper level including the development of insight based on exploration of early development, parental influences and those things *may* come into counselling. In counselling they are brought in to understand a *particular* situation rather than to understand the client him or herself.

One respondent had personal experience of *both* counselling and psychotherapy and made few distinctions between them:

I've had both psychotherapy and counselling as part of my on-going training. I can't say there seems to be that much difference. Some see psychotherapy as synonymous with psychoanalysis but I find it difficult to make that link. Counselling doesn't go as deep as psychotherapy. Psychotherapy is a bit of a status thing as well. No-one really knows, unless you're a psychodynamic therapist – then you know! But there are other sorts of psychotherapy, transactional analysis and so on, I don't know really, the distinctions are blurred.

❏ Differences between counselling and other sorts of conversation

If there were conflicting reports about what counselling and psycho-therapy were, then it would seem reasonable to try to define the boundaries of counselling in another way. To this end, we asked respondents what the differences were between counselling and *other* sorts of conversation. If counselling is a discrete activity (as opposed to, for example, simply talking things over with a friend), it seems reasonable that those who do it should be able to distinguish between simply 'talking' about something and 'doing counselling'. One respondent saw the difference in terms of *structure* – the counselling relationship was a more structured one than the more informal conversation:

The only difference that I can see is in their formal structure. If things can be achieved by talking to your friends in the pub, then that's fine, whereas counselling usually has some sort of formal structure involved. It is also a professional relationship in the sense of a counsellor and client where the counsellor is paid to counsel or listen.

Other respondents described the differences in terms of the *roles* played out by the participants in counselling:

In counselling you would expect that one of the people has a problem, a dilemma that they are facing and that tends to be the focus of the interaction, whereas the other person is seen as a counsellor, helper or listener. In a normal conversation that state of affairs might apply but it might also not apply and there may just be small talk about any aspect of the person's life. If you build on that definitional difference, the more professional the counsellor, or the more formalised the counselling, the greater the difference would be between the helper and the helpee in terms of power, status and so forth. For example, if I go along to a friend of mine and talk about work or home problems, I won't feel guarded about status or power or being exposed psychologically because in that relationship it is guided by the principles of friendship or collegial relationships. On the other hand, if I found that I had to attend a marriage guidance counsellor, for example, I would find that rather uncomfortable. At least to begin with. And I would be very aware that I was the one with the problem and that he or she would be the person with the fix-it solution.

For another respondent, the two types of interaction were often blurred. It was sometimes difficult to say what the difference was between counselling and 'ordinary conversation':

I think that it is a difficult question because sometimes an ordinary conversation turns into counselling and a counsellor may use coun-selling skills in their conversational life. I also think that counselling skills can enhance conversation and, perhaps thinking as we talk about this, counselling is a specific form of conversation. I think sometimes the differences can be small and that initial sessions with clients can be conversational.

On the other hand, another respondent was very clear about the differ-ences and saw them in *contractual* terms:

Counselling has very specific parameters. There is a contract, you know how long you will meet and so on. It is a very specific type of conver-sation. And although some of the skills and things the counsellor may be demonstrating are similar to other conversations it is very *inten-tional.* It is not two-way as in other conversations. The focus in coun-selling is very much on the client. It is intentionally focused.

❑ People who do counselling

If counselling is something to be considered as a therapeutic option by nurses, it is important to know what sorts of people *do* counselling. Should they be *qualified?* Should they be 'professionals', and so on. There were various responses to this sort of question:

Essentially anyone can do counselling. But for the most part it tends to be either professional counsellors or people who have traditionally had a counselling role, such as doctors, nurses or priests.

People do counselling who are interested in other people and who are prepared to spend time with them, supporting them. Anyone could, in that respect, do counselling, whereas in the more formal type of coun-selling – the formal helping agencies – you get the doctors and the social workers. Then there are the people who set themselves up as professional counsellors.

I think that counselling could be done by anyone but is more likely to be done better by someone who has had the opportunity to develop specific skills and who has been able to explore some of his characteristics and things like warmth, genuineness, etc. However, it is likely that many people already possess those qualities and therefore are better helpers than people who do not. I think there is a danger in saying that counselling is the preserve of counsellors because that relates it directly to training and I am not sure there is any evidence to demonstrate that training really does make a difference.

Most of the above respondents took the 'anyone can do counselling' line. Others, however, wanted counselling to be more formalised and for counsellors to be trained:

People who [do counselling] are qualified counsellors, although there may be people who have not done a proper certificate or diploma but who do counsel from experience. There are elements of counselling and counselling skills that occur in a lot of caring conversations that are carried out by health care professionals. It would be wrong to counsel somebody without their permission and without a contract because of counselling's potential power.

❏ What counselling can be used for

If counselling is a therapeutic activity, it seems important to know what counselling can be used for. These responses were drawn from a number of sources within the transcripts:

There are a whole range of practical difficulties that can be helped by counselling, such as difficulty with study skills and getting into higher education, through to things like depression following bereavement, or neuroses or mental illnesses. There has been an expansion in the profession of counselling in recent years – you often get the situation where someone calls themselves a professional counsellor on the basis of a range of qualifications which carry no guarantee as to the likely effectiveness of that counselling.

❏   **The structure of counselling**

One respondent discussed the use of counselling in terms of its *structure* and of how little or much the counselling relationship needed to be structured.

> It can be used on a daily basis or on an informal basis with contacts with colleagues and people you are attached to. I guess this is the more informal type of counselling. Then there are the more professional settings – tutors to students for example, when you have to make yourself approachable to the students. That needs a little bit more thought. Some of the people who are tutors are therefore focusing on academic issues, others are there for all aspects of the student's life. Perhaps a middle path is necessary here: where tutors are prepared to listen to what is going on outside the student's immediate academic arena.

Another talked of 'formalised' counselling (as opposed, presumably, to informal or 'friendly' counselling):

> There is the more highly formalised counselling situation – counselling people, getting paid to do it, perhaps being part of a team helping GPs, psychiatrists, etc. You may be a practitioner in a psychiatric unit or other care setting. All of these different situations are ones in which some form of counselling might be called for.

Another respondent made this distinction between 'formal' and 'informal' approaches to counselling more explicitly:

> There are at least two types of counselling: the informal, ordinary, unspectacular way of helping and the more professional side of things. I find that the phoniness you meet sometimes – the tilted head, the voice changing, may be a result of the training. I find that off-putting. What I need when I discuss something with somebody else is a gut reaction – a more spontaneous reaction. I would not approach a stranger for that. I would need to know the person was genuinely interested in me.

Yet another respondent talked of the difficulty of training counsellors and of the paradox between 'being spontaneous' and 'being a professional':

> The spontaneous part of counselling is very, very difficult to train at all. It has to do with people knowing their limitations and their likes and dislikes. As you professionalise something there is the tendency to make things more special, more detached from the real side of a relationship. Something gets lost. There is a risk of losing the spontaneous side of the interaction.

Others saw the value of counselling as lying within the process of helping people to become more responsible for themselves and re-exercising some control over what happens to them:

It can be used to enable people to examine specific problems or life situations which they would like resolved or changed. To enable them to make the best use of resources, to examine relationships, to make choices, to discover the choices available to them. To help them become more responsible for themselves and to use that responsibility over their own lives. To enable them to feel more in control of their situation. To enable them to be in a relationship with a counsellor which will enable them to learn about themselves. And to make those discoveries in a situation which, although it may be uncomfortable, is safe.

It can be used to enable people to problem-solve, to identify sources of discomfort or stress and it can be used to alleviate problems of living – everyday problems of living such as anxiety and general feelings that people have of being outside. It can also enhance basic communication. It can also be used, perhaps, inappropriately. It can be used as a disguise for basic disciplinary measures and it can be highjacked to disguise commercial activities such as beauty counsellors, financial counsellors, etc.

Some respondents felt there was a tension between health professionals offering counselling and counselling being viewed as a 'treatment'. It was seen as essential that becoming involved in counselling should be a voluntary activity on the part of the patient or client:

I don't think there is ever a should – this person should see a counsellor. If they are not ready and they don't want it, then there is no point. I very much believe in people's rights to live their own life the way they want and not have counselling. When somebody is going through a traumatic experience then there are all sorts of problems that are unresolved particularly when they do not have other people in their lives to talk to. Even when people do have lots of other people counselling is quite different. Family and friends will not talk to you in the same way. Counsellors are impartial and will not necessarily just go with you. Friends will not want to upset you whereas counselling can be more penetrating and challenging – which friends will not always be – unless they are special friends. Any sorts of problem – mid-life crises, what's it all about – those sorts of issues can be addressed in counselling.

❏ When counselling should not be used

Respondents talked about when counselling *should not* be used – contraindications to counselling. These were wide ranging and are reported below:

> It shouldn't be used as a habit or for recreational purposes. I have seen some people who seem to be addicted to it. It becomes a substitution for normal human intercourse and sometimes peoples' motives are poor for going into it in the first place – such as group counselling as a place to pick up women.

> There may be a danger that a vulnerable person could be exposed psychologically or abused – using the term broadly. If you were, for example, attracted to a person of the opposite sex, or the same sex, that may infect the situation if you had a lot of contact with them. As a counsellor you need to be pretty solid, you need to know what you are doing and your integrity is not going to be called into question. You have to be seen as being detached but that's not a word that rests easy, you have to be comfortable in your own skin – whatever people say to you, you're not going to be tempted to abuse the relationship. Those things relate more to the professional dimension than to the ordinary side.

Sometimes the issue was an ideological one. It was noted by one respondent that the prevailing philosophy in counselling is the 'client-centred' one in which the client is *always* encouraged to find his or her own solutions to his or her problems and in which direct, prescriptive intervention on the part of the client is usually eschewed:

> It may depend on the type of counselling the counsellor wishes to adopt. To adopt a non-directive approach with people, where it is patently obvious that you should be making suggestions, is very wasteful; I think there are lots of people who seek out help who want a direction and to keep throwing it back on them and ask them to make every decision is sometimes inappropriate. People are pretty good at problem-solving and are likely to respond much better to the non-directive approach but there are people who find it difficult to make any decisions and then it is appropriate to make more concrete suggestions as to what they may do.

Sometimes, the fact that counselling was not a panacea was noted and it was made clear that counselling had very definite limitations:

> There may be situations where the problem cannot be solved in your head – and I'm thinking about lack of money, serious illness, unem-

ployment – those sorts of things. Counselling may help but some of those very serious problems aren't ones that can be solved. On these emergency situations that we see on the TV – kids drowning, accidents and things – it's amazing how quickly counselling services are set up. And yet what most normal people would be is in a state of shock at that time, and its seems likely that only afterwards people need counselling – not immediately afterwards.

Sometimes the client-centred approach, referred to above, was seen as limited, and one respondent called for a much wider approach to be used:

When the counsellor has motives other than to help the client: when the counsellor is in a situation in which he himself ought to take responsibility for the situation, either because of former responsibilities for it or when not to do so would cause undue pain to the client – such as when you are in situations in which people steadfastly avoid giving advice by trying to be Rogerian – when the best thing would be to tell the person what to do. I recognise that in counselling you would tend to avoid that but sometimes it would be more appropriate. I think John Heron's (1990) material on prescriptive and informative interventions is quite helpful in that way.

Reference was sometimes made to the fact that counsellors always seemed to 'be available' after national disasters:

I think I would also disagree with those who feel that the presence of counsellors at disasters is probably inappropriate. You get a vision of therapeutic vultures; perhaps when people are in extreme distress they need time to be distressed. Because counselling is not a universal panacea for the human condition.

If someone doesn't want counselling, then they shouldn't be 'forced' to have it. I don't think it's a good idea for some person in authority to say you're going to have counselling and that's it. Counselling is often used to mean counselling people in their work or students but that's not the way I mean it.

❏ The advantages of counselling

Various advantages of counselling were identified by the respondents. One respondent identified its *economic* advantages:

It can help you over an immediate crisis or problem. If you are upset you often can't see a way out of a predicament. It's a cheap relative to psychoanalysis or psychotherapy. It is also widely available. A counsellor will give you time in a way that a doctor won't. And for an atheist like myself, a priest is not really an alternative. For a religious person, a priest may be the most appropriate person as the problem may have a spiritual content.

Others found other advantages but these were often *qualified* in various ways, suggesting that with the various advantages also came other disadvantages:

It can be pretty cheap – a cheap way of helping people. The less formal types of counselling perhaps allow the person who needs the help to maintain some dignity and integrity in the whole process and it's not like going to your doctor or going to a psychiatrist because your whole life is falling apart – it's sort of more acceptable to society. You can say to people I'm going for some counselling but it is more difficult to say I am mentally ill. There is a greater willingness for people to take counselling on board as acceptable.

[Counselling helps one to have] the opportunity to have a safe situation in which one explores options and choices – particularly where some of those choices may be frightening or where some disclosures of some aspects of one's self may be a presentation of self that one wouldn't want seen elsewhere. If I am looking at a side of myself that I don't want to show to people in every day life but I need to understand, then I may need the confidentiality of a counselling relationship in order to do that.

The opportunity to have another head, another mind focusing on the problems the individual is struggling with.

❑   The disadvantages of counselling

There were also clearly identified *disadvatages* to counselling. Again, these were quite wide ranging:

It can mislead people into thinking it's a solution, when in fact a real solution may be a material change in the person's circumstances which the counsellor can do nothing to effect. There are a lot of charlatans in counselling. When there is money changing hands the counsellors may have more interest in prolonging the sessions. It is a straightforward market relation sometimes. And like all market relations the profit is a motive and not a human need. The other thing is, it is just another way of accommodating oneself to what may be a horrible situation and a better response may be a political one.

One respondent had doubts about the purported practice of teaching student nurses counselling skills as part of their nursing training – arguing that counsellors needed some maturity and some life experience in order both to help the client and to take care of themselves:

> One of the things which is true about counselling is that is has become reified – it has become elevated to a supernatural status – particularly in nursing. So much so that every curriculum document must have an element of counselling in it. My feeling is that many of the students that I have dealt with are anywhere between 17 and 22 and I do believe that if you're going to be a good counsellor you need to have more life experience as it will help you to put things in perspective. It seems that some courses are expecting to put these young people into counselling and turn them out as mini-counsellors in any arena. I don't think that this is realistic and this is one of the problems as the thing has become more popular. So you have people coming out of courses who will, I think, have done all these hours of counselling training but these are not underpinned by the years of experience that are needed to be a good counsellor.

Other disadvantages were also noted:

> There is the potential opportunity to abuse other people's vulnerability. People do enjoy having power, as experts over people who are very vulnerable, and I think this is something to guard against.

> For the client perhaps, they may feel that it doesn't supply them with any answers. The process can be seen as rather slow or even traumatic.

> For the counsellor the disadvantages are that it opens you to an awareness of another person's pain that you may have to avoid due to the situation you are in. And perhaps it can make you weary of other people's distress.

❏ Applications of counselling in nursing

Respondents talked of how counselling could or could not be used in nursing as part of a range of nursing skills:

> Nurses should be trained in a wide range of counselling techniques. The practical problems that clients face need skilled intervention and this is true in both mental health and somatic medicine. Quite often nursing interventions can be unskilled and tactless and if it changes that then it

will be a useful tool. Because nurses deal every day with other people, especially those people who may be ill and their relatives who may be waiting there with them, counselling training is essential. Those nurses will need certain attitudes and skills to do the job well. They will need to be able to listen to people very carefully and to use the information that they gather from patients and families to drive their nursing assessment of patients. They need to convey to people an attitude of helpfulness but not in a condescending way. They need to be able to help patients and families to deal with the awfulness of death, dying, bereavement, loss, trauma, and anything that the counselling course can offer nurses to help these people is to be encouraged. However, we shouldn't overload the dice. Lots and lots of nurses are being asked to deal with horrible life events in patients' and families' lives with limited support, with limited extra training and no core support mechanisms at work in the organisation to deal with stress.

Again, a respondent returned to the theme of *age* and of the need to be cautious about training nursing students to early in their careers:

I would reiterate the point that it is nonsense to take on 17-year-olds – adolescents – and then force them to have these counselling skills. I think that to be a good counsellor these people have to have some personal experience to ground and contextualise the work that they do and if people wish to undertake counselling skills training it should be done after a very solid foundation of professional experience. And people should at least be in their mid 20s. That is a rough and ready guide. Obviously there are some very mature 18-year-olds and there are some very immature people in late adulthood.

Nurses can utilise basic counselling skills in nursing interactions. Patients often complain of not being listened to or of wanting to talk to somebody. I think the full therapeutic hour has its place in probably a limited number of settings. However, that reason can be used to justify avoidance of encountering patients in any more than a perfunctory manner. I think also some areas of nursing need to embrace a rational basis to their business otherwise those areas of nursing will become very vulnerable. I'm thinking of community psychiatric nursing in particular, if the only activity for which there is a perceived rationale is depot medication, and that places those nurses in a position of potential extinction. Also it makes interactions more purposeful and perhaps it also improves the nurses' use of self by making them more self-aware.

Another respondent referred to the wide range of ways in which counselling or counselling skills could help in nursing contexts:

Counselling skills and listening skills are helpful in any type of helping relationship. When you go to a patient in the morning and say how are you? and being open to the answer – that can help. So I think in almost any interaction the nurse can work much more therapeutically. However, there is much more scope for counselling itself, for example, with a patient who has had an operation – anything where a patient wants to talk about something in more depth. This should be set aside from other nursing duties and the nurse should be able to make it clear that this is a counselling relationship. It is astonishing there is so little available. We are a collection of mind, body, emotions, etc. and it is the mind which we do not deal with very much.

These interviews give examples of the ways in which practising nurse-counsellors and trainers feel about one aspect of the interpersonal skills field. Many of the features of effective counselling – the ability to listen, the ability to focus your attention on the *other person's* problem, and so on – are all related to a more general interpersonal skill – that of being able to relate to patients in a helpful way. However, as we shall see, the term 'interpersonal skill' is by no means clear cut.

■ Interpersonal skills in nursing: the background

During the past 20 years or so, interpersonal and communication skills training has become an important facet of nurse education (Kagan, 1985; Macleod Clark and Faulkner, 1987; Burnard, 1989b). There are many problems connected with learning to be interpersonally skilled. Some of these stem from the fact that the term 'interpersonally skilled' is not clearly defined. In the first part of this chapter, we have explored *counselling* as one example of the use of interpersonal skills in nursing, but the field and its definitions are by no means clear.

In the study to which we now turn, our aim was to try to spell out more clearly what the term 'interpersonally skilled' meant for a group of experienced nurses. This was an attempt to identify the attitudes and/or behaviours that described such an interpersonally skilled person from a nurses' perspective, rather than by adopting a theoretical framework and description from the literature on the subject. The study outlined below describes one method of exploring what is a very complex and disparate field.

■ Approach to the problem

Kelly's personal construct theory and its use as an approach in research was outlined in Chapter 2. The version of the repertory grid technique offered here is a straightforward and practical application that seeks to identify one group of nurses' perceptions of the types of personal construct that constitute 'interpersonal effectiveness'. We tried to identify an 'ideal type' of interpersonally skilled person.

❏   Method

We carried out a survey of 21 trained, professional nurses who were all students on a postgraduate university course. The sample can thus be described as 'opportunistic' (Field and Morse, 1985) in that it was a sample of people who could articulate views and were readily available to the researchers. The limitations of such a sample are acknowledged, and more work would need to be done in order to further validate the adequacy of our findings.

The nature of the Kellyian approach emphasises personal perspectives, and the need to generalise to other groups is not necessarily a condition of this type of descriptive and qualitative research (Field and Morse, 1985). In other words, this is a description of these nurses' perceptions at this time. If we wanted to design interpersonal skills training courses on the basis of these findings, we would have to replicate this study with each new group of nurses in order to identify *their* perceptions and *their* training needs. This approach is in line with the current emphasis on student-centred and negotiated approaches to adult learning (Knowles, 1986; Brookfield, 1987).

The repertory grid procedure in this instance was guided by the one described by Honey (1979). We asked our respondent group to elicit eight bipolar constructs by using six people (the 'elements') that they had identified and could be categorised as follows:

- two people whom you perceive to be interpersonally skilled
- one person you perceive not to be interpersonally skilled
- one person who fits in between these two
- yourself as you are at the moment, and
- yourself as you would like to be (ideal self).

We then asked respondents to consider the six people in terms of their own set of constructs and to rate these people on a scale of 1–5.

■   Analysis of the content of the grids

In order to explore the content of the elicited constructs, we used the method of content analysis, following the procedure suggested by Stewart and Stewart (1981) and described earlier in the book. You will recall that this entailed writing all of the constructs onto small index cards and then sorting these into a small number of similar content areas. The following categories emerged:

- personal qualities
- disposition towards others
- the person's relationship towards self and others
- communication skills, and
- miscellaneous.

We then reported these initial findings back to our respondents and discussed our results with them. This discussion with the respondent group helped us to check on the accuracy of our analysis of the constructs. Comments and suggestions made by the respondents implied that some reorganisation needed to be done. We did this on the grounds that the following categorisation system had greater clarity and more readily conveyed the respondents' perceptions.

Following our discussion with the respondent group, we revised the category system as follows:

- personal qualities (personal characteristics that describe parts of the individual's personality)
- disposition towards others (how the individual thinks and feels about others)
- communication skills (specific skills possessed by the individual)
- disposition towards self (how the interpersonally skilled person thinks and feels about himself), and
- miscellaneous (other attributes that could not be categorised in the above scheme).

A quantitative analysis of the way in which the constructs were distributed in each of the labelled categories was carried out and is illustrated in Table 6.1.

Table 6.1   The distribution of constructs within the five-category scheme (n = 21)

Category	Number	Percentage
Personal qualities	96	57
Disposition towards others	21	12.5
Communication skills	19	11.5
Relationship to self	18	10.5
Miscellaneous	14	8.5
TOTALS	168	100

■ Secondary analysis

Because we asked respondents to rate a 'self' and an 'ideal self' on their own construct set, we were able to examine their perceptions of their own interpersonal effectiveness. To do this, we used a rating scale where 1 lay at one end of the construct and 5 at the opposite end, with 2, 3 and 4 being degrees in between.

To explore the relationship between the 'self 'and 'ideal self', we looked at the structure within the grid scores for each individual respondent. Specifically, a simple difference score (Bannister and Mair, 1968; Honey, 1979) was computed. In Figure 6.1, the pattern of different scores that emerged from 20 of the 21 informants can be seen. One of the informants was unable to complete this aspect of the analysis because of time constraints.

SUMMARY STATISTICS	
Mean	10.68
Standard deviation	4.68
Range	3–21

Figure 6.1   Summary of difference scores for each of the respondents (n = 20).

We found that all the respondents reported a shortfall in their perceptions of their interpersonal performance by calculating the difference between the 'self' and 'ideal self' elements. However, the size of difference between these two elements for a number of respondents suggests that many of the group perceived a significant variation between their actual interpersonal performance and their preferred interpersonal performance, the mean difference score being 10.7.

This finding implies that the respondents rate themselves severely because they perceive themselves as not highly skilled in the interpersonal domain; they have identified their own need for more training. The range of difference scores (3–21) suggests, however, that not everybody viewed themselves so harshly. It is notable that the differences that emerged were always in one direction, which pointed up deficits in their performance. This is, perhaps, not surprising. Typically, however, it is likely that the notion of an 'ideal self' will invoke the idea that this type of self is one to be aimed at and one rather better than the actual self. Relating the 'self' and 'ideal self' was an approach used by Rogers (1951) in psychotherapy.

This particular approach to the problem of identifying the meaning of the term 'interpersonally skilled' has produced three main findings:

1. It has enabled the researchers to identify more general trends in the group's perceptions.
2. It has picked up individual variations in the pattern of self-assessed interpersonal effectiveness.
3. It shows how the researcher can assess and monitor changes following interpersonal training both in the individual and in the group.

In these respects, the repertory grid method as used here provides a flexible yet structured research instrument and has enormous potential for everyday use in the field of interpersonal skills training workshops.

■ Making sense of the results

Perhaps the most interesting finding of this small study is the large number of constructs which were classified as personal qualities. This was by far the largest category. Examples include:

'helpful...never available'
'genuine...deceiving'.

It would seem that the nurses in this study think of *personal qualities* as the most important distinguishing features of interpersonally skilled people. If this finding can be replicated on a larger scale, questions about the 'micro-skills' approach to training interpersonal skills must be addressed. The social skills approach mentioned earlier is a good example of this technique. The implication here is that there is a need to pay more attention to those personal qualities that enhance interpersonal skills and effectiveness. However, the issue of whether or not such qualities could be taught must remain for the moment an interesting and taxing question.

Confusion also remains about whether or not nurses or other helping professionals bring these personal qualities with them into the work setting or whether they are developed during a process of professional socialisation. If the latter is true, we must consider how these qualities are to be cultivated and evaluated. If the former case applies, why has there been such an immense emphasis on interpersonal skills training in nurse education over the last 20 years or so? If nurses already possess some of the essential qualities to make them interpersonally skilled, perhaps much of this training is redundant! A great deal of research will have to be carried out in this area before we can make decisions about these issues.

The second largest category, 'disposition towards others', contained constructs about the person's attitude towards other people and seemed to link with the personal qualities of the previous category. These did, however, emphasise the social interaction with other people. Examples here included:

'approachable...distant'
'empathic...critical'.

The third largest category enclosed constructs which referred specifically to communication skills. A key theme here was the notion of an effective listener. In fact, other sorts of interpersonal intervention were rarely mentioned. This also raises interesting questions about what it is we mean when we talk of 'interpersonal skills'. Examples from this category included:

'listener...bad listener'
'good verbal skills...unclear speech'.

In the next category, we included constructs which referred to the person's relationship with themselves. Examples here included statements about the person being self-aware, for example:

'acceptance of oneself...lack of acceptance of oneself'
'open...preoccupied with self'.

It is significant, too, that the concept of self-awareness was identified by so few of the respondents.

In the last, 'miscellaneous', category we included a range of other constructs which were difficult to classify under the category framework. Some of the constructs here appeared to be very idiosyncratic and not easily related to the other categories. Examples in this category included:

'credible...lacks credibility'
'good personality...shy'.

■ The importance of personal qualities

It is particularly notable that this 'qualities' issue was also one that emerged out of the study of nurses' perceptions of caring (described in Chapter 2). The consistency between the two studies seems to support the idea that therapeutic nursing relationships are more to do with how people feel about and perceive each other than about particular sets of skills. This is interesting when we consider how much attention is often paid to the skills element of interpersonal training in nursing programmes.

The nurses in this study felt that the nurse's personal qualities were of *particular importance* in the interpersonal relationship. However, we must also note that personal qualities have been described by Carl Rogers (1967, 1983) as indispensable qualities for therapeutic change. Rogers argued that these qualities *must* be present if a person is to be helped in therapy. The qualities that Rogers describes are:

- warmth and genuineness
- empathic understanding, and
- unconditional positive regard.

■ Summary

This chapter has identified a range of approaches to interpersonal skills. It has also discussed two studies exploring counselling in nursing and the meaning of the term 'interpersonally skilled nurse'. We see this as a necessary stage in trying to identify a baseline for planning training and education in the field of interpersonal skills. In the next chapter, we consider basic communication skills in nursing: listening and simple counselling techniques.

■ Further reading

Bottorff, J.L. and Morse, J.M. 1994 Identifying types of attending: patterns of nurses' work image. *Journal of Nursing Scholarship*, **26**(1):53–60.
Bulmer, C.A. 1994 Maximum insight with minimum dependence: brief therapy in psychiatric nursing. *Professional Nurse*, **9**(9):621–5.
Gleber, J.M. 1995 Interpersonal communications skills for dental hygiene students: a pilot training program. *Journal of Dental Hygiene*, **69**(1):19–30.

Chapter Seven

Basic communication and counselling skills in nursing

So far, we have highlighted the importance of the relationship between the nurse and patient. We have explored some of the research which looks at the concept of caring and some of the research on nurses' interpersonal and communication skills. We now want to explore in more depth some of the types of skill which are essential for the nurse in a counselling situation. We maintain that the skills of counselling are also those needed by all nurses as effective communication skills. If you can counsel well, you probably communicate well.

■ Basic communication skills

❏ Attending and listening

Listening and attending are by far the most important aspects involved in the counselling process. The best counselling is that in which the nurse only *listens* to the other person. Unfortunately, most of us feel a need to talk, and it is the nurse's 'overtalking' that is least effective. If we can train ourselves as nurses to attend closely to what patients are telling us, and really listen to them, we can do much to help them. However, we need to be able to discriminate between the two processes of attending and listening.

❏ Attending

Attending is the act of really focusing on the person who needs help. We need to make ourselves deliberately aware of what the other person is saying and of what he or she is trying to tell us.

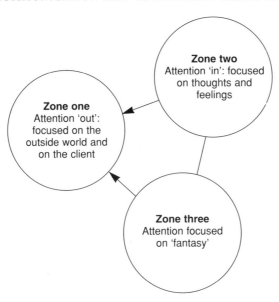

Three possible zones of attention

❏ Listening

Listening is the process of 'hearing' the other person. Given the wide range of ways in which one person tries to communicate with another, this is further evidence of the need to develop the ability to offer close and sustained attention, as outlined above. Three aspects of listening are noted in the diagram. Linguistic aspects of speech refer to the actual words that the client uses, to the phrases they choose and to the metaphors they use to convey how they are feeling. Attention to these is useful, as metaphorical language can often convey more than the more conventional use of language (Cox, 1978).

Paralinguistics refer to all those aspects of speech that are not words themselves. Thus, timing, volume, pitch and accent are all paralinguistic aspects of communication. Again, they can offer us indicators of how the other person is feeling beyond the words that they use. Again, however, we must be careful of making assumptions and slipping into zone three, the zone of fantasy. Paralinguistics can only offer us a possible clue to how the other person is feeling. It is important that we check with the client the degree to which that clue matches with the client's own perception of how he or she feels.

Non-verbal aspects of communication refer to 'body language': the way that the client expresses himself through the use of his body. Thus facial expression, use of gesture, body position and movement, proximity to the nurse and touch in relation to the nurse all offer further clues about the client's internal status and can be 'listened' to by the attentive nurse.

Again, any assumptions that we make about what such body language 'means' need to be clarified with the client.

There is a temptation to believe that body language can be 'read', as if we all use it in the same sort of way. This is, perhaps, encouraged by works such as Desmond Morris's (1978) *Manwatching*. Reflection on the subject, however, will reveal that body language is to a large degree dependent on a wide number of variables: the context in which it occurs, the nature of the relationship, the individual's personal style and preference, the personality of the person 'using' the body language, and so on. It is safer, therefore, not to assume that we 'know' what another person is 'saying' with his body language but again to treat it as a clue and to clarify with the client what he means by his use of it. Thus it is preferable, in counselling, to merely bring to clients' attention the way they are sitting, or their facial expression, rather than to offer an interpretation of it. Two examples may help here. In the first, the nurse is offering an interpretation and an assumption:

> I notice from the way that you have your arms folded and from your frown that you are uncomfortable with discussing things at home.

In the second example, the nurse merely feeds back to the client what she observes and allows the client to clarify his situation:

> I notice that you have your arms folded and that you're frowning. What are you feeling at the moment?

Levels of listening

The skilled nurse learns to listen to all three aspects of communication and tries to resist the temptation to interpret what she hears. Three levels of listening may be identified:

Linguistic aspects:
- special phrases
- use of metaphors
- the words that are spoken
- content
- coherence

Paralinguistic aspects:
- accent on particular words or phrases
- 'ums' and 'ers'
- fluency
- timing
- volume
- pitch

Non-verbal aspects of communication
- facial expression
- the way the client uses gesture
- touch

- body position
- proximity to the nurse
- body movement
- eye contact

	NURSE	CLIENT
Level 1	Hears words	Talks
Level 2	Maintains 'free-floating' attention	Talks and experiences some empathy
Level 3	Hears words, maintains 'free-floating' attention and notes her own feelings	Feels listened to and understood

Figure 7.1   Three levels of listening.

Figure 7.1 offers a framework for thinking about listening. The first level of listening refers to the idea of the nurse merely noting what is being said. In this mode, neither client nor nurse are psychologically very 'close', and arguably the relationship will not develop very much. In the second level of listening the nurse learns to develop 'free-floating' attention. That is to say that she listens 'overall' to what is being said, as opposed to trying to catch every word. Free-floating attention also refers to 'going with' the client, not trying to keep the client to a particular theme but following the client's conversation wherever it goes. The nurse also 'listens' to the client's non-verbal and paralinguistic behaviour as indicators of what the client is thinking and feeling. Faced with this deeper level of listening, the client feels a greater amount of empathy being offered by the nurse. The nurse begins to enter the frame of reference of the client and to explore his perceptual world. She begins to see the world as the client experiences it.

In the third level of listening, the nurse maintains free-floating attention, notices non-verbal and paralinguistic aspects of communication but also notices her own internal thoughts, feelings and body sensations. As Rollo May (1983) noted, it is frequently the case that what the therapist is feeling, once the counselling relationship has deepened, is a direct mirror image of what the client is feeling. Thus the nurse sensitively notices changes in her self and gently checks these with the client. It is as though the nurse is listening both to the client and to herself and carefully using herself as a sounding board for how the relationship is developing. Watkins (1978) has described this process as 'resonance' and points out that this process is different from that of empathising:

> Rogers says that empathy means understanding of the feelings of another. He holds that the therapist does not necessarily himself experience the feelings. If he did, according to Rogers, that would be identification, and this is not the same as empathy. Resonance is a type of identification which is temporary. (Watkins, 1978)

The use of resonance needs to be judged carefully. It does not involve interpreting or offering a theory about what the client is feeling. It does offer a particularly close form of listening which can make the client feel listened too and fully understood. It is notable, too, that in these circumstances the client will often feel more comfortable with periods of silence as he struggles to verbalise his thoughts and feelings. Arguably, he allows these silences because he senses that the nurse is 'with him' more completely than at other levels of listening. The net result of this deeper level of listening is that a truly empathic relationship develops. The client feels listened to, the nurse feels she is understanding the client and a level of mutuality is achieved in which the two are communicating, both rationally and intuitively.

Use of 'minimal prompts'

Whilst the nurse is listening to the client, it is important that she shows that she is listening. An obvious aid to this is the use of what may be described as 'minimal prompts' – the use of head nods, 'yes', 'mm', and so on. All these indicate, 'I am with you'. On the other hand, their overuse can be irritating to the client, particularly, perhaps, the thoughtless and repetitive nodding of the head – the 'dog in the back of the car' phenomenon! It is important that the nurse, at least initially, is consciously aware of her use of minimal prompts and trys to vary her repertoire. Very often, such prompts are not necessary at all. Often all the client needs is to be listened to and appreciate that the nurse is listening, without any need for further reinforcement of the fact.

❏ Attending, listening and the nurse

The attending and listening aspects of counselling are essential skills that can be used in every nurse's job. The skills are clearly not limited only to use within the counselling relationship but can be applied in other interpersonal exchanges. An advantage of paying attention to the development of these particular skills is that becoming an effective listener not only makes for better counselling practice but also enhances interpersonal effectiveness and self-awareness.

■ The client-centred approach to counselling

Perhaps the most frequently used approach to counselling is that known as *client-centred counselling*, the founder of which is generally recognised as being Carl Rogers, the American psychotherapist and humanistic psychologist (Rogers, 1951, 1983). Client-centred counselling eschews the giving of advice and asks of the counsellor that he or she simply helps the client to find *his* way towards a solution to his problems. The client-centred approach is based on the idea that we all have a potential for personal growth and that, given the time and space, we can usually find our own solutions to our own problems. Indeed, it is sometimes argued that we are the *only* people who can find such solutions. More can be found on the client-centred approach in Burnard (1994).

It might further be argued that *nursing* has, until recently, been *prescriptive.* That is to say, nurses in the past tended to 'tell' patients what was or was not good for them. This is in exact contrast to the client-centred approach. We wondered, therefore, to what degree nurses would see themselves as client-centred in their practice. To that end, we devised a study using the Nelson-Jones and Patterson Counselling Attitude Scale (Nelson-Jones and Patterson 1975). It is claimed that the scale helps to measure 'client-centredness'.

Table 7.1   Distribution of the sample (n = 142)

Grade	Number
District nursing students	24
Health visiting students	24
Staff nurses (general nursing)	22
Professional nurses *	20
Community psychiatric nursing students	21
Qualified community psychiatric nurses	12
State enrolled nurses	10
Practice nurses	9
TOTAL	142

* The nurses in this group comprised those who were over 30 years of age, with more than 4 years experience of nursing in a position of responsibility. This group was made up of nurse tutors, nurse managers and senior clinical nurses.

■ Attitudes to counselling in nursing

In the present study a total of 142 nurses were asked to complete and score the Nelson-Jones and Patterson Counselling Attitude Scale (Nelson-Jones and Patterson, 1975). The distribution of that sample is illustrated in Table 7.1. The sample was a opportunistic one (Field and Morse, 1985) in that respondents were taking part in counselling skills workshops run by one of the authors (PB). The instrument was administered at the beginning of the workshop and before any discussion of counselling or counselling skills had taken place.

■ The research instrument

The Nelson-Jones and Patterson Counselling Attitude Scale is a 70-item questionnaire. Respondents are asked to read each item and to respond by indicating that they agree with, disagree with or could not decide about each item. Examples of statements from the questionnaire are as follows:

- The nurse should ask questions only when he does not understand what the client has said.
- If a client wants to discontinue counselling, he should be allowed to do so.
- The more information the nurse has about the client prior to the counselling interview, the better he will be able to understand the client.

The scale was devised by Nelson-Jones and Patterson out of work on other scales which attempted to measure client-centred attitudes. The test–retest reliability of the scale was found to range from 0.88 to 0.91 for three different groups of respondents (Nelson-Jones and Patterson, 1975). The issue of validity was less clear in that Nelson-Jones and Patterson attempted to assess content validity by asking nurses – who were committed to the client-centred approach – to complete the questionnaire. While all of those nurses achieved high scores on the questionnaire, some disputed the degree to which all of the statements reflected a client-centred attitude (Nelson-Jones and Patterson, 1975).

In this study, the nurses were asked to fill in the questionnaire. They were then asked to check the answers to each of the questionnaire items against the scoring system provided by the authors of the scale. The results of that scoring are said to reflect the degree or otherwise of the respondents' client-centredness. Thus a score of 70 on the questionnaire (correct answers to each of the questionnaire items) indicated an extremely client-centred attitude according to the scoring system. Lower scores indicated a lesser tendency towards client-centredness. No problems were identified in administering or marking the questionnaire.

■ Analysis and findings

The range and mean scores were calculated for the total sample and for each of the sub-groups. Table 7.2 offers a comparison of the range and mean scores of each of the groups and the range and mean scores for the total sample.

The mean scores appear to fall into three groups:

1. Health visiting students, professional nurses and community psychiatric nursing students who all scored over 40 on the scale. These mean scores were all beyond the midpoint score of 35 on the attitude scale. It should be noted, however, that *individual* scores varied considerably within the groups.
2. District nursing students, staff nurses and qualified community psychiatric nurses who all scored between 35 and 40 on the scale. In these groups one group had a mean score at the midpoint of the attitude scale and the other two scored just over the midpoint. Individual scores varied considerably.
3. State enrolled nurses and practice nurses who scored 33 and 31 respectively. In these groups, neither mean score was above the midpoint on the attitude scale, although individual scores, again, varied.

The picture to emerge from the group as a whole was that there was only a slight tendency towards a client-centred attitude (mean score = 39). There was, however, a wide range of scores achieved throughout the group.

Table 7.2   Comparison of range and mean scores (n = 142)

Nursing group	Sample size	Range	Mean group score
District nursing students	24	24–47	37
Health visiting students	24	32–59	45
Staff nurses	22	25–50	35
Professional nurses	20	35–67	47
Community psychiatric nursing students	21	24–63	44
Qualified community psychiatric nurses	12	27–50	37
State enrolled nurses	10	27–45	33
Practice nurses	9	22–37	31
TOTALS	142	22–67	39

■ Discussion

Perhaps the most notable finding was the lack of a tendency towards client-centredness in the nurses completing this questionnaire. Given the increasing emphasis on individualised care and the encouragement of patient autonomy, this is disappointing. It suggests that some nurses may still be more comfortable with an interpersonal style that is prescriptive rather than facilitating. This further supports the findings of our studies into nurses' perceptions of their own interpersonal skills, discussed in the next chapter.

However, some of the groups of respondents show encouraging tendencies towards a client-centred approach. Notably, the health visiting students, professional nurses and community psychiatric nursing students showed more of a tendency in this direction than did other groups. While it may be the case that professional nurses, through their increased nursing experience, have come to value a less directive approach, the student group findings are less easy to explain. One possibility is that students tend to discuss such things as interpersonal skills training as part of their courses, and this may have influenced their completion of the questionnaire. On the other hand, if this is the case, it is difficult to explain why the district nursing student group did not score in a similar fashion.

It is notable that no particular difference can be noted between the scores of the general nurses and those of community psychiatric nurses and community psychiatric nursing students. It may have been imagined that psychiatric nurses, given the emphasis on interpersonal skills training prescribed by the 1982 syllabus of training (ENB, 1982), would value the client-centred approach more highly.

On the other hand, it is notable that the community psychiatric nursing students scored more highly than their qualified counterparts. There are at least three possible explanations here. One is that the 1982 syllabus *has* influenced more recently qualified nurses towards a client-centred approach. Another is that those students are studying interpersonal skills on their courses and are thus more aware of the client-centred approach. A third possibility is that such students are more idealistic about the nature of interpersonal relationships than are nurses-in-practice. What is noticeable from the findings is the tendency for nurses-in-practice to score lower on the attitude scale than those who are students (with the exception of the group labelled 'professional nurses').

The tendency for students of various sorts to score more highly than their qualified counterparts may also be accounted for in terms of their being *in training* and thus away from the pressures of the 'real world' of nursing. In the clinical situation nurses frequently have to focus on getting through the work, while students may be able to be more reflective about what they *should do* in their relations with others.

Furthermore, it is notable that the professional nurse group tended to score more highly than other groups. Given that this group was made up of nursing managers, tutors and senior tutors with some experienced ward sisters, it is possible that their score on the scale has been influenced to some degree by the lack of clinical contact of some members of the group. Perhaps the more removed a practitioner becomes from direct patient care, the greater a tendency he or she has to describe nursing actions from the 'ideal' standpoint.

The clinical component of nursing carries with it responsibility, the need to make swift and important decisions and calls for direct response to a whole range of human problems. The clinical practitioner is thinking on her feet, while students and those at one remove from the clinical setting can afford, and are encouraged to be (Ashworth and Morrison, 1989), more reflective about the ideal role.

Two other points are also relevant here. It may be that nurses who work under pressure and have to make many 'instant' decisions will also tend to be more prescriptive in their responses to others. It may be that the client-centred approach, is, by its reflective nature, more time consuming and therefore less immediately attractive as a form of nursing response. Nor may it be the most efficient way to work in a busy clinical setting.

The second point is that, because of the problem of having to respond to so many requests from patients, relatives and colleagues, the nurse may adopt a prescriptive role as a means of defence against anxiety. This explanation may account for why the enrolled nurse and practice nurse groups scored low in terms of client-centredness. Both groups have close contact with large numbers of patients and both work in busy (if different) settings. Arguably, too, the practice nurse group may perceive their role as being legitimately more prescriptive in nature.

All of these issues raise questions about the relevance of the client-centred approach in nursing. While it clearly has a place in psychotherapy and counselling (Rogers, 1967), it may be that a variety of both client-centred and more prescriptive approaches to nurse–patient interaction are the norm. Perhaps, too, they are *required* in certain clinical settings. This chapter raises various questions about the nature of the nurse–patient relationship, but more research remains to be carried out in this complicated field.

■ Summary

This chapter has briefly examined basic communication and the client-centred approach to counselling. In one study in this chapter, nurses were asked to define and talk about counselling. In the other study, we explored nurses' attitudes towards the client-centred approach and found that nurses generally did not show a marked tendency towards it. We have discussed some of the reasons why this may be the case. In the next chapter, we move on to explore a wider range of communication skills using Six Category Intervention Analysis.

■ Further reading

Neubauer, J. 1995 The learning network: leadership development for the next millennium. *Journal of Nursing Administration*, **25**(2):23–32.

Parker, D.L., Webb, J. and D'Souza, B. 1995 The value of critical incident analysis as an educational tool and its relationship to experiential learning. *Nurse Education Today*, **15**(2):111–16.

Rakoczy, M. and Money, S. 1995 Learning styles of nursing students: a 3-year cohort longitudinal study. *Journal of Professional Nursing*, **11**(3):170–4.

Stevens, J. and Crouch, M. 1995 Who cares about care in nursing education? *International Journal of Nursing Studies*, **32**(3):233–42.

Stockhausen, L. 1995 The clinical learning spiral: a model to develop reflective practitioners. *Nurse Education Today*, **14**(5):363–71.

Chapter Eight

Six Category Intervention Analysis and nurses

In this chapter, we report a study that used a theoretical framework known as Six Category Intervention Analysis (Heron, 1986). We describe the Six Category framework, outline a methodology for the study and discuss some of the practical and theoretical implications of the main findings. Some suggestions for future research and training in the field are offered.

■ Six Category Intervention Analysis

Six Category Intervention Analysis (Heron, 1975, 1986) developed out of previous work by Blake and Mouton (1976). It is a conceptual framework for classifying varieties of effective interpersonal intervention between practitioners and clients. Heron's category analysis is a theoretical analysis, and we could uncover no reference to any empirical studies that predated the development of the analysis, nor could we find any later published studies which used the analysis to guide research in this domain.

However, Six Category Intervention Analysis system has been widely used at the Human Potential Research Project, University of Surrey as a tool for training people in using communication skills. Many of those courses are attended by nurse teachers and nurse practitioners and have been recommended by the National Boards as suitable for those who wish to develop their interpersonal skills (Nicolas and Gooderham, 1982).

The six types of intervention in the Analysis are further sub-divided under the headings 'authoritative' and 'facilitative'. Authoritative interventions are those which permit the practitioner to keep some degree of control over the relationship and include the prescriptive, informative and confronting categories. In contrast, facilitative interventions are those that ensure that the locus of control stays with the client; these include the cathartic, catalytic and supportive categories. Figure 8.1 and Table 8.1 identify and describe these categories.

AUTHORITATIVE CATEGORIES	FACILITATIVE CATEGORIES
1. Prescriptive	4. Cathartic
2. Informative	5. Catalytic
3. Confronting	6. Supportive

Figure 8. 1 Authoritative and facilitative categories.

Heron's analysis may be compared with Blake and Mouton's (1976) original Intervention Category Analysis, which was made up of the following categories:

1. acceptant
2. catalytic
3. confrontation
4. prescription, and
5. theories and principles.

The scheme devised by Heron appears to have enhanced the internal logic of the category analysis. He has removed the 'theories and principles' category and added others. It is useful to note also that Blake and Mouton's attention was focused on interventions made in management, whereas Heron's concern is with interpersonal interventions. The *purpose* of the two sorts of analysis is different. It is significant, too, that Blake and Mouton's analysis was intended for use in a fairly specific context, while Heron claims a much wider range of application for his analysis.

Table 8. 1 Synopsis of the Six Category Intervention Analysis

Category	Nature of the intervention
1. Prescriptive	To offer advice, make suggestions
2. Informative	To offer information
3. Confronting	To challenge
4. Cathartic	To enable the release of emotion
5. Catalytic	To 'draw out'
6. Supportive	To encourage or validate

A number of claims about the Six Category Intervention Analysis are made by Heron. He asserts that the category analysis offers an exhaustive range of therapeutic interventions. Furthermore, he claims that the inter-personally skilled person is one who can move appropriately and freely between the various categories as a means of guiding therapeutic action. According to Heron, no category is more or less important than any other category. Paradoxically, however, he argues that catalytic interventions form a 'bedrock' type of intervention that may serve as the basis for effective communication and counselling. He also offers the view that because we live in a 'non-cathartic society' (Heron, 1977b), where the overt expression of strong emotion is not highly valued, the cathartic category will tend to be less frequently and less skillfully used by many practitioners.

Fielding and Llewelyn (1987) note that there are different degrees of resistance to the overt expression of emotion within the UK, influenced by culture. Others may not perceive cathartic release as being of such importance. George Kelly, for example, in acknowledging the need to 'look forward' in life rather than to look back at past experiences, says, 'the only valid way to live one's life is to get on with it' (Kelly, 1969).

The category analysis is focused at the level of *intention*. In other words, it does not pick out a number of specific verbal behaviours but tries to direct the user's intentions in making interventions in therapeutic settings. Thus it is not a mechanical, behavioural training device but a means of helping the user to distinguish between a range of varied therapeutic (and, by implication, non-therapeutic) interventions.

The question remains, however, of the degree to which researchers can have access to people's intentions and whether or not people can remember their intentions after the event! The word 'intervention' is used here to describe any verbal or non-verbal statement or behaviour that the practitioner may use in the therapeutic relationship. The word 'category' is used to denote a range of related interventions.

In the context of psychiatric nurse education Hammond (1983) suggested that category analysis could be employed in two ways: (1) as a means of interpreting nurse–patient interventions, and (2) as an aid to the nurse during counselling sessions. Bond and Kilty (1983) described the application of the category analysis for use in peer support groups. Dryden (1985) also discussed the use of the analysis in teaching counselling skills to 'non-psychologists'. The use of the category analysis in interpersonal skills training and counselling skills development had been described elsewhere (Burnard, 1985).

■ Earlier research using Six Category Intervention Analysis

We completed two previous studies using a ranking schedule based on the category analysis, to ascertain students' and trained staff's perceptions of their interpersonal skills (Burnard and Morrison, 1988; Morrison and Burnard, 1989a). In one of the studies (Burnard and Morrison, 1988), 93 trained nurses completed questionnaires to provide us with details about their perceptions of their interpersonal skills. The following rank order emerged:

1. supportive
2. informative
3. prescriptive
4. catalytic
5. cathartic, and
6. confronting.

In the above overall ranking, item 1 represents the category that respondents felt *most* skilled in using and item 6 the category they felt *least* skilled in using. Our study of student nurses' perceptions yielded a similar response pattern, and many particulars of the differences between the two studies can be obtained from the reports cited above.

■ Further developments in Six Category research

The rest of this chapter is concerned with our most recent attempt to confirm the findings of those previous studies. On this occasion, we elected to use an alternative method of collecting data based on the category analysis described here. A rating scale was used in this study because it allowed greater flexibility of analysis than did the ranking schedule.

The study described here built on previous work on the Six Category approach. We wanted to find out whether or not there was a consistency in the way nurses viewed their interpersonal skills in terms of Heron's analysis. If consistency is present, we may be more confident in using our results to develop training methods, educational policy, assessment techniques and further research.

■ Methodology

This was essentially a quantitative survey. However, our approach was guided by the principle attributed to George Kelly: 'If you want to know something about someone, ask them, they might just tell you' (Epting, 1984). Thus our objective was to ask the nurses in our sample to tell us how they perceived their own interpersonal skill levels, while the category analysis served as a framework for making sense of these perceptions. We used a convenience sample (Field and Morse, 1985) of 117 trained nurses who attended counselling skills workshops run by one of the present authors (PB). These nurses were from the fields of general, psychiatric and community nursing.

■ Procedure

Following a period of introduction and familiarisation with the category analysis, the nurses in each case were invited to take part in the study by completing a rating scale (Figure 8.2).

CATEGORY	NOT SKILLED				VERY SKILLED
1. Prescriptive	1	2	3	4	5
2. Informative	1	2	3	4	5
3. Confronting	1	2	3	4	5
4. Cathartic	1	2	3	4	5
5. Catalytic	1	2	3	4	5
6. Supportive	1	2	3	4	5

Figure 8.2   Six Category rating scale.

■ Analysis level 1

Once the rating scales had been completed, we drew up a matrix consisting of rows and columns in which each row represented a respondent and each column represented a category of the analysis. From this matrix, we were able to calculate mean rating scores for each of the categories, and from these we were able to rank order the six categories in terms of the dimension 'least skilled – most skilled'. These findings are illustrated in Table 8.2.

Table 8.2   Mean rating and rank order of the six categories

Type of intervention	Category	Mean rating	Rank order
Authoritative	Prescriptive	3.75	3
	Informative	3.94	2
	Confronting	2.37	6
Facilitative	Cathartic	2.81	5
	Catalytic	3.30	4
	Supportive	4.23	1

Each respondent had to rate the six category items to correspond with how skilled they perceived themselves to be in their dealing with patients in a professional nursing setting.

❏ Results

Our findings were as follows. The category that was identified as the one the respondents felt most skilled in using was the supportive category (mean rating score 4.23, rank order 1). The informative category was in second position (mean rating score 3.94, rank order 2). Third was the prescriptive category (mean rating score 3.75, rank order 3). The catalytic category was ranked next (mean rating score 3.30, rank order 4), followed by the cathartic category (mean rating score 2.81, rank order 5). The confronting category was in last position (mean rating score 2.37, rank order 6). This rank order mirrors exactly the rank order of our previous study of trained staff's perceptions of their interpersonal skills in terms of the six categories (Burnard and Morrison, 1988; Morrison and Burnard, 1989a).

❏ Discussion

This study further confirmed the suggestion that nurses percieve themselves to be more skilled in being supportive, informative and prescriptive and less skilled in being catalytic, cathartic and confronting. In our previous work (Burnard and Morrison, 1988; Morrison and Burnard, 1989a) we made some suggestions as to why these trends may be found so consistently. We do not intend to repeat these arguments again in this chapter but offer the following list of factors that may help to throw some light on these results:

- The organisational culture (Sathe, 1983) in hospitals may work against the development of a facilitative style of interpersonal relationships between nurses and patients.
- The 'facilitative' approach takes time. Nurses may feel that they do not have time to spare to develop relationships that involve being catalytic, cathartic and confronting.
- Catalytic, cathartic and confronting approaches involve an 'investment of self' that may be emotionally draining. Some nurses may (1) not want to make such an emotional investment, and/or (2) not be sufficiently trained in using these methods.
- Nursing often involves practical activities, and nurses may see the job as involving 'getting the work done' (Melia, 1987). This may mitigate against the use of a more client-centred approach to working.
- There has been a considerable emphasis on the 'information-giving' aspect of nursing care (Hayward, 1975; Boore, 1978; Devine and Cook, 1983). This may account for some of the emphasis on the informative category noted in this study. Indeed, some nurses may view their jobs as being more concerned with information-giving than

with being catalytic or cathartic. Other studies have also confirmed the need for patients to be given accurate and appropriate information. For example, Brearley (1990) found that information can help patients to cope with stress, while Wilson-Barnett (1984) noted that information can lessen the intensity of experienced symptoms in illness. Cohen (1981) found that information can help to promote recovery from surgery and Ferguson (1979), in a study of children aged between 3 and 7 years, found that information played a vital role in their preparation for surgery. On the other hand, information-giving also has its limitations as it can *induce* anxiety in some patients (Ziemer, 1983). Leino-Kilpi *et al.* (1993) offer a detailed review of the literature in the field of information-giving in nursing and health care.

- It may be the case that many aspects of nursing practice do not require the use of catalytic, cathartic and confronting skills. The respondents in our studies have offered a general picture of their skills. It may be that catalytic, cathartic and confronting skills are only rarely used or needed. It would seem odd to argue that all six categories are equally frequently required, given their different nature. On the other hand, the person who does not often use certain interventions may also not be very skilled in using them when she has to. This raises complicated questions about the nature and content of interpersonal skills training programmes.

These points should also be reviewed in the light of our findings in Chapter 4 – where we developed a qualitative and descriptive picture of the nurse at work. The two studies complement each other in many ways.

The issue that remains clear is the consistency with which the pattern of response, in terms of the six categories, has recurred. Thus it would seem that for many nurses, the rank order – supportive, informative, prescriptive, catalytic, cathartic and confronting – characterises their perceptions of their own interpersonal skills. These data were also subjected to a secondary level of analysis which we describe below.

■ Analysis level 2

We also analysed the same data set using multidimensional scaling (MDS), which is a set of mathematical techniques for exploring 'hidden structures' in large sets of data (Kruskal and Wish, 1978; Forgas, 1979; Schiffman *et al.*, 1981). These techniques use proximities between any kinds of variable as input. A *proximity* is a number indicating how similar or how different two variables are or *are perceived to be*. The output is a spatial representation, consisting of a geometric configuration of points, rather like those on a map. Each point in the configuration corresponds to one of the variables or items. This configuration reflects the latent or hidden structure in the data and often makes the data much easier to understand. The more similar two variables are perceived to be, the closer they will be in the spatial 'map'. The reverse is also the case: the more dissimilar two variables are perceived to be, the further away from each other they will be.

With this data set, the variables are the Six Category interventions, and our aim was to explore how these were related to each other. In particular, we wished to know if the classification of interventions into (1) authoritative, and (2) facilitative would be confirmed.

There are a wide range of MDS programs and procedures available (Schiffman *et al.*, 1981). The program which we used is Smallest Space Analysis (SSA) (Borg and Lingoes, 1987). Shapira (1976, p. 137) describes this technique in the following manner:

> This analysis provides a geometric representation of the different variables as points in a Euclidean space. The distance between pairs of points in the space correspond to the correlations of the variables. Hence, two points are closer if the correlation between the corresponding variables is higher.

The researcher's task, having laid out this visual representation, is to *interpret* what underlying processes may be at work 'behind' those representations. The process may be compared with looking at a geographical map and trying to identify what the land actually looks like to the traveller.

We used the computer program SSA-1 from the Guttman-Lingoes (Lingoes, 1973) suite of MDS procedures. From the raw data set, this program generated a matrix of coefficients and a visual 'map' as described above. Our task was then to interpret and try to explain the configurations produced in this way. SSA works by initially calculating a series of similarity coefficients between each pair of Six Category items. The matrix of coefficients produced in this way is shown in Table 8.3.

Table 8.3   The matrix of coefficients produced by the SSA procedure

Type of intervention						
1. Prescriptive	0.00					
2. Informative	0.47	0.00				
3. Confronting	−0.20	−0.04	0.00			
4. Cathartic	−0.38	−0.26	0.29	0.00		
5. Catalytic	−0.31	−0.04	0.30	0.27	0.00	
6. Supportive	−0.01	0.19	0.08	0.21	0.02	0.00

A two-dimensional solution was then requested and produced. The accuracy of the representation produced in this form of analysis is measured by estimating its coefficient of alienation. A coefficient of alienation of 0.15 or below is usually taken to be satisfactory. In this case, the coefficient of alienation was 0.07.

The two-dimensional plot of the Six Category items produced in this analysis is shown in Figure 8.3.

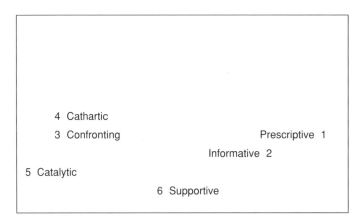

Figure 8.3   Two-dimensional SSA representation of the Six Category items.

It can be seen that the items in the analysis form two distinct groups. The groups formed were of items 1 and 2; and items 3, 4 and 5, with item 6 falling in between these two extremes. Items 1 and 2 are those which referred to more *dispassionate* interpersonal skills, while items 3, 4 and 5 are skills of a more *emotionally charged* nature. A line may be drawn which joins these two groupings, and this line represents a dimension which ranges from an 'emotionally charged' to 'dispassionate' orientation.

The supportive item (item 6), falls within a separate region and is less well described by either of the two poles of this dimension. The central positioning of this item may signify that it is related to each of the two poles of the dimension: thus supportive skills may be either emotionally charged or dispassionate.

❏   **Discussion of analysis level 2**

Initial inspection of the coefficient matrix reveals several interesting points. Both positive and negative relationships between the Six Category items can be seen. This suggests that the area of understanding covered by the rating questionnaire was not perceived by the respondents to be a single unified area.

A closer inspection of the coefficients shows that the negative and positive relationships are orderly. Items 3, 4 and 5 are all interrelated positively to each other, and negatively related to other items. This suggests that these items or interventions are perceived by respondents as being similar skill types. The same is true of items 1 and 2. Item 6, however, has a low and usually positive relationship with all the other items, and is consequently usually related to all other skills. Supportive skills are seen by the respondents to be related to most other interpersonal skills.

The structure of the two-dimensional representation suggesting the two major groups provides little support for the division of interventions into authoritative and facilitative, as described by Heron (1989).

Our analysis suggests a different set of relationships: prescriptive and informative interventions grouped together, confronting, cathartic and catalytic interventions grouped together, with supportive interventions underpinning both of those groups.

The structure provided by the SSA procedure directly challenges that outlined by Heron and suggests that the conceptual framework may need to be revised in the light of these findings. Such a revision may have implications for those in the field of interpersonal skills training and for practitioners in clinical settings.

It would seem from our findings that the nurses in this study perceived themselves to be more skilled in the dispassionate aspects of interpersonal skills and less skilled in the emotionally charged aspects. It is notable, however, contrary to Heron's authoritative/facilitative dichotomy, that the nurses in this study aligned the *confronting* interventions with cathartic and catalytic ones, thus deviating from Heron's original formulation. This may offer an insight into training needs: the aspects of interpersonal skills that require most attention in nursing are those concerned with catharsis, catalysis and confrontation – all of which may be viewed as having a strong *emotional* component.

It is significant that the nurses in our study perceived themselves to be *most skilled* in being supportive, which is the skill that appears to underpin all the others in our analysis. This may offer a starting point for future interpersonal skills training. Rather than the emphasis in such training being on the development of a range of elaborate interpersonal skills, perhaps the basic skill of being supportive is the one that needs to be developed before all others.

❏ Implications

Which types of skill and intervention are *you* good at? Do you avoid emotionally charged situations? Are you confident of your ability to confront other people? Consider how you could further develop your interpersonal skills at work – and at home.

■ Summary

This chapter has described an approach to studying and learning interpersonal skills called Six Category Intervention Analysis. It has also discussed a study of nurses' perceptions of their own interpersonal skills using the analysis and noted that they tended to see themselves as being rather directive in their approach to patients. Few differences were noted between the perceptions of students and those of trained nurses.

■ Further reading

Bateson, C.D. and Coke, J.S. 1981 Empathy: a source of altruistic motivation for helping? In J.P. Rushton and R.M. Sorventino (eds) *Altruism and Helping Behaviour: Social, personality and developmental perspectives*. Lawrence Erlbaum Associates, New Jersey.

Bayntun, L.D. (1993) Setting the scene for experiential learning. *Nursing Standard*, 7(36): 36–8.

Chapter Nine

Nurses and self-disclosure

Self-disclosure is one of the most basic forms of human encounter. When we interact with other people we reveal ourselves to others in various ways and to varying degrees. However, the whole idea of self-disclosure, like the idea of *self*, is a very complicated one. In this chapter, we examine *some* of the issues that influence the process of self-disclosure and attempt to apply these to the work of the nurse.

We disclose ourselves to a number of different sorts of people. A short list of groupings of people might include:

- family
- friends
- colleagues
- nurses and therapists
- other professionals, and
- strangers.

This is not an exhaustive list, but it may help us to focus on the elements of self-disclosure that are particularly relevant for nurses.

❏ Family

At first sight, it may appear that self-disclosure in the family is necessarily high. It seems likely that people will talk to other family members more freely because of the intimate nature of family relationships and because of the amount of time spent with family members. This is especially so when we are young, but as we approach adolescence and young adulthood we begin to expand the range of people we talk to openly.

However, in families, Jourard (1971) noted that people disclose *selectively* to different members of the family. Children, for example, do not tend to disclose equally to both fathers and mothers. Pinkus and Dare (1975) discuss the frequency with which 'family secrets' are uncovered in counselling and therapy. They claim that family secrets can be 'handed down' through families without conscious awareness. They suggest that children often 'guess' at some of the secret issues that parents keep from them and that many of these guesses are accurate. However, as the secrets themselves are never disclosed within the family, the children are inclined to live out those secrets in their own married relationships.

❑   **Friends**

Friends are another group of people with whom we share our thoughts and, unlike families, are to a greater or lesser degree freely chosen. Jourard's work again suggests that people do not disclose equally to both opposite and same-sex friends. It might be imagined that same-sex relationships allow friends to share commonalities of experience that are not shared across the sexes.

However, a number of elements, such as the degree of friendship and the level of closeness and intimacy, may influence the situation. Some people prefer to encourage deep and intimate friendships, while others tend to live on a more superficial plane. Nor is it necessarily the case that friendships are reciprocated in equal amounts. It seems quite possible for one person to want or try to encourage a deeper friendship than the other either wants or is prepared to develop.

❑   **Colleagues**

Colleagues are also people to whom we disclose things about ourselves. The category 'colleagues' is sometimes a large one and might well include people with whom we have close, personal relationships that would almost count as 'friendships' and, in contrast, people we work with but with whom we have little interpersonal relationship. Disclosure to colleagues might often be of the sort that involves offering *information* as opposed to the sort that involves the sharing of feelings, values and beliefs, as may be the case in family or friend relationships. Information can also be withheld from colleagues, and this can mean that the lack of self-disclosure can be used as a means of developing and maintaining control over others. The concepts of 'friend' and 'colleague' may or may not overlap, and this will influence the nature of self-disclosure between these two people.

❏ Nurses and therapists

Counselling and therapy offer a 'formal' means of self-disclosure. Within the boundaries of the professional helping relationship, a person is free to disclose his or her feelings, thoughts, anxieties, doubts, fears, and so on. One of the main aims of counselling and therapy is to encourage people to disclose things about their lives. In this setting, one of the nurse's or therapist's main skills is the ability to help clients to tell *their* story. Counselling and therapy both involve developing a close professional relationship as a way of helping a person with a problem of living. As this relationship develops, the participants will disclose information about themselves. However, the pattern of disclosures is imbalanced – the onus is on clients to take the lead and disclose things about themselves.

Murray Cox (1978) offers a device for identifying the level of self-disclosure in counselling or psychotherapeutic relationships. He distinguishes between three levels of self-disclosure by the client. First-level disclosures, according to Cox, are safe and relatively unimportant ones. Examples of such disclosures will vary according to context but examples might be:

- It took me some time to find your office...
- I had difficulty in parking...
- It took me a long time to get here...

These are civil statements that act as 'feelers' in the relationship and test out the relationship in terms of trust and confidence. The client, it can be imagined, is working out, slowly, whether he or she is able to trust the nurse enough to be able to make more personal disclosures.

Second-level disclosures refer to the disclosure of feelings. Again, such disclosures will depend on the individual and the context of the relationship, but examples of second-level disclosures might be:

- I feel very anxious...
- I'm really angry about that...
- I'm upset when I'm at work...

According to Cox, second-level disclosures will not occur until the relationship between the nurse or therapist and the client has matured sufficiently and the client feels confident and trusts the nurse or therapist. It may be a significant indicator that the relationship has deepened when the client begins to offer disclosures of how he or she is feeling.

Third-level disclosures are those that indicate the really deep, existential concerns of the client, which the client may not have disclosed to anyone before or may have disclosed only to a very small number of people. The clients are often relieved to have told somebody what they have been storing up for a long time. However, they may also be concerned about what the nurse or therapist *makes* of the disclosure. Clearly, to have bottled something up for some time means that the client is unsure about how other people will react.

Third-level disclosures tend to be idiosyncratic and defined by the individual, the relationship and the context. Sometimes they are offered as 'asides' and can be missed by the nurse or the client. For this reason, most of the literature on counselling skills stresses the paramount importance of effective listening (Heron, 1990). Heron suggests that asides be treated as special cases and that the client should be encouraged to repeat them in order to draw out the full importance of them to both client and nurse.

Sometimes third-level disclosures are offered in the form of metaphors. The client may, for example, say 'I never really had a childhood' or 'I am right on the edge, now and there is no turning back…'. Clearly, sensitivity and judgement are required in order to 'make sense' of these types of disclosure. Other third-level disclosures may be more direct and descriptive in nature:

- I've never told my parents that I hate them…
- I've never really loved my husband…

The disclosures made in counselling and therapy may be different from other sorts of self-disclosure. The nurse's role is one of helping in the *formulation* of the disclosures. In many therapy settings, some form of self-disclosure is a central concern. In many cases, the aim is for the client to disclose and, through such disclosure, solve problems, resolve life difficulties and learn new ways of coping.

The role of the professional nurse in a counselling or therapy setting is a very powerful one because of the unequal status of the two participants. Rogers, in the context of counselling, argues that both nurse and client can share a mutual relationship (Rogers, 1967). However, few counselling or therapeutic relationships involve total mutuality and balanced levels of self-disclosure.

❏ Other professionals

As a nurse, you may be called upon to disclose things to a range of other professionals, from managers to social workers and from doctors to the police. While this sort of self-disclosure is usually within fairly narrow boundaries and does not necessarily involve the disclosure of feelings, it may well be facilitated by the formal *roles* played out by the professionals who need information from us.

Those other professionals who are empowered to request information from us usually do so through formal interviews, by the use of specific forms or by other, clearly defined methods. This highly structured process usually allows disclosure without embarrassment. The doctor's role, for example, is made easier for both her and the client by the 'distancing' that the role allows (Myerscough, 1989). It also makes it easier for the patient to be frank and less embarrassed when talking about 'sensitive' issues.

❏ Strangers

The 'stranger on the train' phenomenon has been noted in the social psychology literature (Atkinson *et al.*, 1990). Some people have a tendency to disclose, fairly quickly and fairly deeply, to strangers, apparently because of the helpful effect of telling other people about ourselves and the realisation that both parties are unlikely to meet again. A variant of self-disclosure to strangers may be found in the religious practice of confession. Self-disclosure of this sort is carried out in relative secrecy (usually a confessional) and is usually associated with having a redemptive character. It may also be cathartic in the way that self-disclosure in counselling may be cathartic. The 'stranger' element may be found in the anonymity of the relationship between the confessor and the one confessing.

Another example of disclosing to strangers is that which takes place in the context of the UK's Samaritan counselling service. The Samaritans offer a totally anonymous and completely confidential service to anyone in need of help. Beyond the confidentiality of this service must also lie the need that is satisfied by being able to disclose information on any subject to a complete stranger.

■ Verbal and non-verbal forms of self-disclosure

The forms of self-disclosure discussed in this chapter are all forms of *verbal* disclosure. It is also the case that we disclose ourselves non-verbally (Argyle, 1985) and through the way we dress, the way we present ourselves to others and the countless other ways in which we tell other people who we are. Clearly, too, there are languages through which people communicate but which are not verbal, examples of these being the various sign languages that are used by deaf people.

■ Other factors that affect self-disclosure

The issue of whether or not we self-disclose is not only limited by the question of to whom we make the disclosure. A short list of other factors might include the following:

- the degree to which we are extroverted or introverted
- social norms and expectations
- whether or not we are 'high' or 'low' disclosers
- mood and temperament
- our reading of the social situation at the time
- our desire to communicate or otherwise with another person
- the number of personal problems we perceive ourself to have and the urgency of our need to share them
- the insistence of the other person to have us self-disclose
- the perceived 'pay-off' of self-disclosure
- unconscious factors limiting or not limiting our disclosure, and
- the status of the person to whom we are disclosing.

■ The need to self-disclose

People need to disclose things about themselves. We choose to disclose ourselves to each other in friendships and relationships as a way of enhancing intimacy and of developing reciprocity. Jourard explicitly refers to this when he suggests that 'disclosure begets disclosure' (Jourard, 1964). According to Jourard, the person who discloses him or herself to another person is likely to encourage that person to disclose in return.

It seems possible, however, that some people can be over-eager and disclose too much about themselves too readily. If the person receiving the disclosure feels that the other person is disclosing too much about herself, he may feel that reciprocation is expected, although he may not *wish* to disclose so explicitly. In this case, rather than 'disclosure begetting disclosure', it is possible that disclosure mitigates against mutual disclosure. Usually, the process is incremental and the exchange is evenly balanced – although this may not always be the case.

■ Some problems

Much of the literature on self-disclosure focuses on the positive nature of things. A number of problems might be identified here. First, if people's life experiences vary along with their personality types and their interpretation of their experiences, it seems likely that what constitutes 'deep' self-disclosure for one person will not be so deep for another. It is possible, for example, to imagine that one person will find it easy to disclose factors about his or her family, while another person will not. In the domain of sexuality, the issue becomes even more clouded. The person who takes a liberal view of sexuality may be able to disclose more about his or her sexuality than the person who considers the topic taboo. If there is variation in what might constitute 'deep' disclosure, it is difficult to argue the pros and cons of the *effects* of such disclosure.

Second, we presumably learn about appropriate levels of disclosure as we grow up. There are things, for example, that we would not disclose, at home, to our parents (although this rule might not always apply, either). Then there are things that we might disclose to close friends, to colleagues, to strangers, and so on. All of these variables, in terms of depth and in terms of to whom a disclosure is made, make the topic a difficult one to study.

A third problem involves the person to whom a disclosure is made. There can be no real way of establishing, *a priori*, how the person hearing a disclosure might react to it. The fact that the disclosure *still has to be made* is evidence in itself that the reaction of the 'listener' cannot be gauged. Presumably, if the listener's reaction *could* be gauged, the process of self-disclosure would not be problematic. If we knew beforehand that a disclosure would be favourably met, we would have no hesitation in making it. On the other hand, if we knew for certain that a disclosure would not be favourably met, we would not make it. The fact remains that we simply cannot know in advance what a difference our self-disclosure will or will not make.

Linked to the previous problem is one that involves the discloser. Just as it is impossible to know beforehand how the 'listener' will react to a disclosure, so it is also impossible for the potential discloser to know how *he* or *she* will feel once he or she has disclosed. Traditional wisdom suggests that we might feel better if we get things off our chests. This view, supported through notions of confession and catharsis, indicates that an issue that is disclosed is an issue that makes the person feel better. However, this may not always be the case – sometimes we may disclose things that we later regret.

■ A study of self-disclosure in nursing personnel

The remainder of this chapter is concerned with two studies that replicated some of the work of the psychologist Sidney Jourard. Jourard's work in the field was extensive during the 1960s and early 1970s (Jourard, 1964, 1971). His work has been widely cited in the literature on counselling and psychotherapy, in the literature on caring in the health professions and, perhaps most particularly, in the humanistic psychology literature (see for example Nelson-Jones, 1982; Egan, 1986; Rowan, 1988; Burnard, 1990). In addition, all types of research – particularly the qualitative and in-depth types of study – involve some degree of self-disclosure .

Our interest in Jourard's studies came from our backgrounds in the psychology and mental health fields and manifests itself in a variety of research projects and publications in the area of communication and inter-personal skills (e.g. Burnard and Morrison, 1991; Morrison *et al.*, 1991). We were also impressed by the clarity of Jourard's reporting of his work and by the seemingly straightforward nature of the studies that he had completed. Indeed, as we shall see, that simplicity might be both an advantage and a disadvantage.

The first stage of the study reported here was of a direct replication of a Jourard study from 1961 in which he used a questionnaire to explore levels of self-disclosure in a small group of university students. We were able to replicate his study almost exactly. In the second stage, we used a group of trained nurses to explore other differences in self-disclosure levels.

❏   Stage 1

The initial stage was a replication of Jourard's 1961 study of 25 British, female university students with a mean age of 19.88, ranging from 18 to 25 years. All subjects in Jourard's study were unmarried and were classified as middle class. A 25-item questionnaire was used. Respondents were asked about the level of information that they disclosed to four important people (target persons) in their lives – their mother, their father, their closest male friend and their closest female friend.

Jourard reported that the split-half reliability of the questionnaire had previously been demonstrated with groups of American informants, from which he obtained correlations of 0.9 or higher. In summary, Jourard found that there was a marked tendency for females to disclose more to other females than to males. When comparing his British findings with a comparable sample of American students, Jourard also noted that the American students were generally more disclosing than were the British – they had a higher mean disclosure rating than the British respondents.

The American students also displayed a tendency to disclose more to females than to males. In rank order, the students in the British study disclosed most to their mothers, then to their closest female friends, then to their fathers and lastly to their closest male friends. Overall, Jourard also noted a similarity between the American group and the British group in terms of the relative disclosability of certain questionnaire items to certain target persons.

Our aim was to repeat the British element of Jourard's 1961 study. We wanted to know the degree to which a study conducted 30 years after Jourard's would show similarities and differences in terms of self-disclosure between young female university students. We planned to make a direct comparison between our findings and those reported by Jourard.

We asked 25 female undergraduate nursing students in a UK university to complete Jourard's 25-item questionnaire. The mean age of the group was 19.72 and the range was 17–23 years. This was an opportunistic sample (Field and Morse, 1985) of 25 students drawn from a larger pool of students. All respondents volunteered to take part in the study.

Respondents were asked to complete the questionnaire that Jourard had used in his 1961 study. In a later publication (1971) Jourard reproduced the questionnaire in full and gave permission for the questionnaire to be used in future studies. The questionnaire was completed by reading 25 statements pertaining to items of personal information and then rating the degree to which the respondents felt that they had disclosed those items of information to their mother, father, same-sex and opposite-sex friend. Examples of the items of information in the questionnaire included:

- the food you like best and the way that you like the food prepared
- whether or not you belong to any church, and
- details of your sex life at the present time.

Some minor modifications of the wording of the questionnaire were made in order to suit the sample. An example of one such wording change is as follows. Item 10 of Jourard's questionnaire reads: 'Whether or not you belong to any clubs, fraternity, civic organisations; if so, the names of these organisations'. We changed this to read: 'Whether or not you belong to any clubs, if so, the names of those clubs'. We thought that this would not make a significant difference to the outcome of the study but would make the items easier to understand. All answers to questionnaire items were recorded by the respondents on response sheets. We also asked for details of the respondents' age and sex. All the respondents were female.

Informants were instructed as follows:

We are interested in how much you self-disclose to people that you know. We are replicating a study that Sidney Jourard undertook in 1961 with nurses and want to find out if self-disclosure by nurses has changed or stayed the same. We would be grateful if you would take ten minutes to fill in this questionnaire.

Below is listed a number of items of information about oneself. You are asked to indicate on the special answer sheet the extent to which certain other people know this information about you through your telling it or confiding it to them.

If you are certain that the other person knows this information fully – so that he or she could tell someone else about this aspect of you – write the number 1 in the appropriate space. If the other person does not know this information fully, if he or she has only a vague idea, or has an incomplete knowledge of this particular item, write in 0.

Remember, do not write in a 1 unless you are sure that you have given this information to the other person in full enough detail, that they could describe you accurately in this respect to another person.

You are not required to put your name on the response sheet and you cannot be traced personally or by hospital from your sheet. Also, you are not being asked to disclose any personal information about yourself.

SELF-DISCLOSURE QUESTIONNAIRE ANSWER SHEET

Write 1 in the column if you have disclosed the information in the item, fully, to the person in question. Write 0 in the column if you have not disclosed the information, fully, to the person in question. Please make sure there is a 1 or a 0 in each square.

Item Number	Your mother	Your father	Female friend	Male friend
1				
2				
3				
4				
5				

Figure 9.1   Section from the response sheet completed by respondents.

Once the 25 respondents had filled in their response sheets we were able to calculate the frequencies of response to particular items and the number of disclosures to target persons (mother, father and same- and opposite-sex friends).

Findings from stage 1

The scores outlined here summarise the patterns of disclosure that emerged for this sample of nurses. We examined the relative disclosability of particular questionnaire items for the group. In Table 9.1, it can be seen that, across the group, the same-sex friend achieved the highest number of disclosures and the father figure received the lowest. The mean scores summarise the overall trend, but the range of scores suggests considerable variation within the sample. The mean scores were also plotted against Jourard's reported figures, and this allowed us to make a direct comparison with Jourard's original data.

Table 9.1   Summary of findings from student group (n = 25). (All mean scores have been rounded up)

	Target figure			
	Mother	Father	Same-sex friend	Opposite-sex friend
Overall score	417	316	447	388
Range	5–22	3–22	10–25	6–25
Mean	17	13	18	16

The second level of analysis focused on individual respondents. We were able to identify the total number of disclosures made by each student to each of the four target figures. This allowed us to explore the pattern of disclosure for each student. The pattern is illustrated in Table 9.2.

A few observations may be made about these patterns of disclosure. First, some respondents appeared to disclose quite highly to all four target persons. For example, respondent 21 had a total score of 78 disclosures. The range of those disclosures was 18–21. The total score suggests that, relative to other respondents, she was a high discloser. The narrow range suggests that she was comfortable disclosing things to all four target persons.

On the other hand some respondents appeared to be more selective about whom they disclosed to even though they could also be regarded as high disclosers. For example, respondent 23 had a total score of 73 disclosures, the range of which was 14–25. The total score, again, suggests that she was a high discloser, but she appeared to be much more selective about which target persons she disclosed to. In this particular instance the respondent disclosed only 14 items to her father, while being prepared to disclose all items to her same-sex friend.

Table 9.2   Pattern of individual student disclosures (n = 25)

Respondent	Total number of disclosures	Range	Mean
1	62	8–20	15.5
2	70	15–19	17.5
3	53	6–18	13.25
4	48	4–17	12
5	62	6–25	15.5
6	79	18–21	19.75
7	59	7–25	14.75
8	58	8–20	14.5
9	64	13–23	16
10	66	12–19	16.5
11	80	17–24	20
12	57	11–22	14.25
13	74	14–25	18.5
14	57	13–16	14.25
15	53	10–15	13.25
16	72	7–23	18
17	41	5–17	10.25
18	63	12–20	15.75
19	55	3–21	13.75
20	50	9–21	12.5
21	78	18–21	19.5
22	81	17–22	20.25
23	73	14–25	18.25
24	49	4–18	12.25
25	61	12–19	15.25

In contrast, some respondents, for example, were prepared to disclose *all* items to at least one target person, while others would not disclose certain items to *any* of the target persons. This highlights some of the subtle issues that are at stake in the study of self-disclosure. It is not simply a matter that some people can be designated 'high disclosers' and others 'low disclosers'. It seems from this sort of analysis that at least the following disclosure styles exist:

- there are people who will disclose much to all target persons
- there are people who will disclose much to selected target persons
- there are people who will not disclose much to any target persons, and
- there are people who will disclose a considerable amount to target persons but will not disclose *certain* things.

This type of analysis raises questions about what determines whether or not a person discloses things about him or herself and what factors affect the likelihood of such disclosure. Also, what influences the *context* of disclosure? How do people make decisions about to whom they will disclose certain issues and not others? All of these questions have significance both for those who work in the 'disclosing professions', such as counselling, nursing and psychotherapy, and also for further research into self-disclosure.

❏ Stage 2

In the second stage of the study, we wanted to increase the number of respondents invited to take part in the study and to choose a different type of sample. The aims and sampling procedure in this stage of the study were similar to those used in the first stage, but in this instance 25 senior nurses were selected. They were all female, over 21 years of age and registered nurses. A number of them were married; this was another distinguishing feature between this sample and that used in the first stage of the study. It quickly became apparent that the fact of being married made a difference to the findings since married respondents reported that they counted 'disclosure to an opposite-sex friend' as 'disclosure to husband'.

Findings from stage 2

The findings are summarised in the format used with the student sample – examining the pattern of disclosure with regard to the target persons and exploring the pattern of disclosures for individual respondents (Tables 9.3 and 9.4).

Table 9.3   Summary of findings from senior group (n = 25)

	Mother	Father	Same-sex friend	Opposite-sex friend
Overall score	343	276	295	522
Range	1-24	0-24	1-23	10-25
Mean	13	11	12	21

Target figure

Table 9.4   Pattern of senior group disclosures (n = 25)

Respondent	Total number of disclosures	Range	Mean
1	25	2–11	6.25
2	57	8–19	14.25
3	88	15–25	22
4	48	5–23	12
5	73	11–25	18.25
6	66	13–14	16.25
7	63	8–22	15.75
8	53	9–21	13.25
9	61	5–24	15.25
10	40	1–18	10
11	44	1–24	11
12	55	7–24	13.75
13	42	6–20	10.5
14	71	13–23	17.75
15	81	13–25	20.25
16	59	8–25	14.75
17	67	9–25	16.75
18	42	0–19	10.5
19	50	5–25	12.5
20	64	10–22	16
21	57	10–25	14.25
22	61	12–23	15.25
23	28	1–19	4
24	84	18–23	21
25	47	6–21	11.75

Again, it will be noted that there was a variety of response patterns across the group. Disclosure was often highest to opposite-sex friends, which may be explained by the fact that an unspecified number of the respondents were married. The range of scores across the respondents varied considerably, some respondents disclosing nothing to one of their target persons and others disclosing all items to one of their target persons. On the other hand, some respondents had a narrower range of disclosures, which helps to confirm the idea that there may be 'high disclosers' and 'low disclosers'. Further research may usefully explore the factors that could account for these differences.

❏   **Differences between student group and senior group**

Comparison of Tables 9.1 and 9.3 reveals differences in the types of disclosure revealed by both sample groups. Table 9.5 shows the mean score differences between the two groups for disclosures to target persons in each group.

Table 9.5   Total numbers of disclosures for the sample groups

	Students (n = 25)	Senior respondents (n = 25)
Number of disclosures	1568	1436
Mean scores	392	359

First, the students tended to be more willing to disclose to their mothers and same-sex friends than did the senior respondents. Generally, the senior respondents were willing to disclose more to opposite-sex friends than were the students, and less inclined to disclose to the other target persons, but this style of disclosure may be explained by the fact that many of the senior respondents were married.

Second, in both groups there was scope for considerable variability in the disclosures reported. For example, a number of the senior respondents claimed to be prepared to disclose all of the items on the instrument to their opposite-sex friends, while one senior respondent claimed that she disclosed nothing to her father.

Third, the students in this study were generally more disclosing than were the senior respondents (as measured by the total number of disclosures for each of the sample groups across all target persons). This difference is illustrated in Table 9.5. However, this sort of crude measurement may disguise the individual, idiosyncratic scores that lie beneath it. On the other hand, there may be implications for differences of disclosure between age groups.

❏ Disclosing particular items

A further analysis of one of the student data sets was undertaken to explore Jourard's idea of 'disclosure begetting disclosure' a little more closely. We felt that it was important to explore the *types* of information that people might disclose to one another. This younger group of respondents was also chosen for more detailed analysis because the earlier research studies also focused on younger respondent groups.

The self-disclosure questionnaire contained a number of different sorts of item, ranging from those concerned with what sports a person might take part in to those about sexual behaviour. It seems likely that people will, overall, be more forthcoming about certain issues than others. The following list shows the items, in rank order, according to how often they were scored by respondents as having been disclosed to one or more of the target persons. In other words, a high-ranking item is one that was frequently disclosed and a low-ranking item is one that was not frequently disclosed. This list gives an indication of the degree of ease or difficulty that respondents felt in disclosing aspects of themselves to significant others. A score of 0 would indicate that an item was not disclosed by any respondent to any of the target figures. A score of 100 would indicate that an item was disclosed by all respondents to all target figures. In practice, the pattern of responses was never as extreme as this, and it is interesting to note that there was fairly even distribution of the items throughout a range from 41 to 80.

❏ Rank order of questionnaire items

In this list, questionnaire items are rank ordered according to the number of times they were cited as being disclosed by respondents across all target persons. Thus the higher the ranking, the more frequently respondents reported disclosing this item. In addition, the mean number of disclosures for each item is reported. Table 9.6 offers an overview of what respondents were prepared to disclose and the order of the likelihood of their disclosing any particular item.

❏ Comment

Other questions can be asked about both the validity of this sort of investigation and about the whole idea of exploring self-disclosure. If this sort of questionnaire aims at identifying those who do self-disclose and those who do not, we might be tempted to imagine that those who could state that they were prepared to disclose all of the items in the questionnaire might be said to have self-disclosed fairly comprehensively. However, the issue seems to be far more complicated.

Sitting with a stranger and disclosing all of the items on the questionnaire would necessarily mean that we disclosed ourselves to that person. The business of self-disclosure would seem to be much more complicated than simply telling other people certain facts about ourselves. While we can acknowledge that certain facts are likely to be more 'private' than others and, therefore, more difficult to disclose, it does not follow that if we disclose a considerable number of 'difficult' issues, we have disclosed 'more' of ourselves.

■ Summary

Jourard, in his studies, has suggested that 'disclosure begets disclosure'. He develops this proposition out of the studies in which he made considerable use of instruments, such as the one that we have described and used here. Therefore his proposition is based on the prior proposition that 'self-

Table 9.6 Rank order of disclosed items in student study

Number of disclosures	Mean score	Item
87	3.48	Whether or not you belong to any church, if so, which one and the usual frequency of attending
86	3.44	The sports you engage in most, if any, e.g. swimming, tennis, etc.
84	3.36	What you like to do most in your spare time at home, e.g. read, sports, go out, etc.
84	3.36	The places that you have travelled to, or lived in during your life – other countries, towns, etc.
79	3.16	Any skills you have mastered, e.g. arts and crafts, painting, sculpture, etc.
78	3.12	Whether or not you drink alcoholic beverages: if so, your favourite drinks – beer, wine, etc.
76	3.04	The kinds of music that you enjoy listening to most, e.g. popular, classical, folk-music, opera, etc.
75	3.00	The kind of party or social gathering that you enjoy most
73	2.92	The names of the people in your life whose care and happiness you feel in some way responsible for
71	2.84	The kind of future you are aiming towards, working for, planning for – both personally and vocationally, e.g. marriage, family, professional status, etc.
68	2.72	Whether or not you belong to any clubs, if so, the names of those clubs
67	2.68	An exact idea of your regular income (if a student, of your usual combined grant, allowance and earnings, if any)
66	2.64	Whether or not you have any favourite spectator sports, if so, what these are, e.g. football, tennis, etc.
66	2.64	The foods you like best, and the ways you like food prepared, e.g. rare steak, etc.
63	2.52	Your usual and favourite spare-time reading material, e.g. novels, non-fiction, science fiction, poetry, etc.
56	2.24	Whether or not you have been seriously in love during your life before this year, with whom, what the details were and the outcome
55	2.20	Whether or not you know and play any card games, e.g. poker, bridge, etc.
51	2.04	Your thoughts about your health, including any problems, worries or concerns that you might have at present
46	1.84	How you feel about the appearance of your body – your looks, figure, weight – what you dislike and what you accept in your appearance, and how you wish you might change your looks to improve them
45	1.80	The personal deficiencies that you would most like to improve, or that you are struggling to do something about at present, e.g. appearance, lack of knowledge, loneliness, temper, etc.
43	1.72	Your problems and worries about your personality, that is, what you dislike most about yourself, any guilt, inferiority feelings, etc.
43	1.72	Whether or not you are now involved in any projects that you would not want to interrupt at present – either socially, personally, or in your work; what these projects are
42	1.68	The details of your sex life up to the present time, including whether or not you have had or are now having sexual relations, etc.
40	1.60	Whether or not you presently owe money, if so, how much and to whom
23	0.84	What your political sentiments are at present – your views on political parties and policies

disclosure equals the amount of personal things that one person will tell another about him or herself'. In this chapter, we have questioned the validity of this position. If the position does turn out to be open to question in this way and if self-disclosure might mean more than how much one person is prepared to tell another, the 'disclosure begets disclosure' proposition may also be open to question. The proposition might more correctly be stated as 'people who are prepared to reveal things about themselves are more likely to encourage other people to do the same'. Despite these criticisms, the process of telling other people about ourselves is likely to influence our relationships with others in professional settings.

■ Further reading

Bauer, J. 1994 Proactivity... a personal habit that deals with self-awareness and being committed to our own values. *Journal of Post Anesthesia Nursing*, **9**(4):272, 271.

Fleming, J. and Strong, J. 1995 Self-awareness of deficits following acquired brain injury: considerations for rehabilitation. *British Journal of Occupational Therapy*, **58**(2):55–60.

Malkin, K.F. 1994 A standard for professional development: the use of self and peer review; learning contracts and reflection in clinical practice. *Journal of Nursing Management*, **2**(3):143–8.

Sutherland, J.A. 1995 The Johari Window: a strategy for teaching therapeutic confrontation *Nurse Educator*, **20**(3):22–4.

Chapter Ten

Learning to care and communicate

How do we learn to care and communicate? One approach is through the use of our own experience via experiential learning methods. In this chapter, we explore the notion of experiential learning and report a study of nurses' perceptions of it.

Experiential learning is the process of learning by direct, personal experience. It can be contrasted with 'book' learning and with learning through lectures. However, those distinctions are not quite fine enough. Weil and McGill describe four 'villages' as an approach to defining different types of experiential learning (Weil and McGill, 1989):

1. **Village one: The assessment and accreditation of 'prior' experiential learning**

   Essentially, the people in this village view experiential learning as learning from life experience and learning that can be 'totted up' to enable adults to gain exemption from certain degree and diploma courses. In the UK, for example, nurses who have not gained 'first' degrees can sometimes gain entrance to master's degree courses by virtue of their previous personal and professional experience.

2. **Village two: Experiential learning and change in higher and continuing education**

   In this village, experiential learning is often tied closely to adult learning theory and the notion of developing learner-centred approaches to teaching and learning.

3. **Village three: Experiential learning and social change**

   In this village, experiential learning is a radical process concerned with helping people to change the circumstances in which they find themselves.

4. Village four: Personal growth and development

Here, the emphasis is on the individual's learning processes, and the people of this village are often aligned with the humanistic school of psychology. It is arguable that it is this 'village' that has most strongly influenced the development of experiential learning in nurse education.

Weil and McGill's argument, then, is that we can learn much from *all* approaches to experiential learning – from the political aspect of it, from the adult learning approach, as well as from the personal growth and development aspect.

Experiential learning, then, describes the following:

1. a set of teaching/learning methods, and
2. an attitude towards learning.

■ Research into experiential learning

Although a great deal has been written about the theory of experiential learning and the fact that it has been advocated as an approach well suited to the teaching of nursing skills, very little research is available on the topic. The study described here forms part of a larger study into the theory and practice of experiential learning in nurse education. The aim of the study was to identify how nurse educators perceive the concept of experiential learning as it applies to their work as nurses educators.

■ Method

A group of 12 nurse educators were interviewed. The main focus for the interview was their views of experiential learning. This was a purposive sample (Fink and Kosecoff, 1985). Bogdan and Biklen (1982) describe such a sample as one which is designed to best facilitate the emergence of relevant theory. The sample was made up of a variety of educators from England and Wales (and one from Australia) who were mostly teachers of psychiatric nursing, the others being general nurse teachers. All claimed to use experiential learning methods in their educational practice. The sample included lecturers, senior tutors and nurse tutors.

A semi-structured interview schedule was used to guide the interviews, which lasted for between 30 and 45 minutes each. The interviews were tape-recorded and the tapes were later transcribed. All participants took part in the interviews voluntarily, and each was offered an explanation of the purpose of the study in line with Reason and Rowan's (1981) argument that researchers in the social sciences should be explicit in stating their intentions when setting out to do research.

■ Analysis and key findings

Content analysis (Carney, 1972) was then used to identify thematic patterns in the transcripts. This method of analysis, as used here, helped to explore only the overt content of interviews; it cannot hope to identify latent content. Overt content refers to the meanings in written or spoken data that are clear and unequivocal, no attempt being made to look for hidden assumptions. Latent content refers to hidden or personal meanings that are usually present in all speech and writing, yet which are extremely difficult to access during data analysis.

All the transcripts were read through and then categories were identified from the questions that had been asked. The broad category headings that were used can be seen in Figure 10.1.

- Definitions of experiential learning
- Examples of experiential learning methods
- Examples of learning methods other than experiential ones
- Advantages of the experiential approach
- Disadvantages of the approach
- Evaluation methods

Figure 10.1 Category headings following content analysis.

The transcripts were then re-read in order to determine what each of the interviewees had said under each of the headings. In this way, a series of sub-headings was generated from the data. During this process, a number of categories were 'collapsed' to form clearer, more discrete sets of categories. Reliability checks were undertaken by inviting a colleague to read through a number of transcripts and identify her perception of the categories. Agreement was then reached on 'core' categories.

Using these sub-headings, it was then possible to read through the transcripts again and note to what degree there was agreement or disagreement about definitions, methods, and so on, between the interviewees. A grid was drawn up which showed the categories/sub-categories and frequency of response to those categories by respondents (Field and Morse, 1985). An example of part of that grid is illustrated in Figure 10.2. This procedure enabled the researcher to quantify the strength of any particular responses by counting its frequency and then assigning it a rank order. Each transcript was re-examined and the presence or absence of an interviewee's response to a particular category/sub-category was noted. No limitation was placed on the number of categories that could be identified within a particular category from a particular transcript.

	DEFINITIONS		
	Learning from past experience	Learning from present experience	Whole life experience
Interviewee 1	6		
Interviewee 2			6
Interviewee 3		6	

Figure 10.2 Example from the analytical grid.

■ Perceptions of experiential learning

❏ Definitions

The first category identified in the study was that of definitions of experiential learning. Table 10.1 illustrates the sub-categories that were generated from the transcripts, along with the frequency with which they were cited by the educators and placed in rank order.

Table 10.1   Definitions of experiential learning (n = 12)

Definitions	Frequency	Rank order
1. Learning through doing	8	1
2. Affective learning	4	= 2
3. Whole life experience	4	= 2
4. Learning from past experience	3	4
5. Learning from present experience	2	5
6. Role play	1	6

It is notable that a range of definitions was offered – there was no general agreement about what constituted experiential learning. The range varied from the most frequently cited definition (learning through doing) to definitions which accented various dimensions of life experience: the whole of life, past life experience and present life experience – the 'here and now'. One interviewee saw experiential learning as being synonymous with role play, an interesting finding, since role play is more usually seen as an example of an experiential learning method rather than as a definition (see the section below on methods).

Some of the interviewees (n = 4) admitted that they found experiential learning difficult to define. This is a curious statement given that all of the respondents claimed to be using experiential learning methods in their day-to-day teaching and had acknowledged a strong interest in the concept prior to the research! If they were using it extensively, it is not too much to expect them to be clear in their own minds about what it is and how it works. This paradox may suggest a limitation in the method used in the study. Perhaps a period of observation in the learning environment with some of the nurse tutors and students would help to clarify the situation.

The variety of ways of defining experiential learning is interesting as it suggests that it may be defined by different people in different ways. If nurse educators vary in their definitions of experiential learning it seems likely that learners will perceive experiential learning in different ways. On the other hand, it is difficult to know to what degree differences of definition are important, as there was much less difference of opinion about what constituted experiential learning methods (see the next section).

❏ Experiential learning methods

The next category to be identified was that of experiential learning methods. Interviewees were asked to identify what they would describe as examples of experiential learning methods. Table 10.2 illustrates the sub-categories that were generated in this section.

Table 10.2   Examples of experiential methods (n = 12)

Experiential learning methods	Frequency	Rank order
1. Reflective activities	9	1
2. Role play	8	2
3. Practical activities	7	= 3
4. Structured group activities	7	= 3
5. Humanistic therapies	5	5
6. Games and simulations	3	= 6
7. Altered states of consciousness	3	= 6
8. Learning aids	2	= 8
9. Physical activities	2	= 8

A majority those interviewed (n = 9) identified activities that involved reflection on experience as being an example of experiential learning methods. Some identified role play as a method (n = 8), while others (n = 7) talked of practical activities such as getting learner nurses to feed each other or practising making beds with the learners as 'patients'. Some also described structured group activities of the type described by Pfeiffer and Jones (1974 and ongoing) as examples of experiential learning methods (n = 7). These usually involved the group undertaking a well-defined activity, followed by a period of reflection and sharing of the experience. A number of respondents (n = 7) also referred to a wide range of humanistic therapies as examples of experiential learning methods. These included transactional analysis, Gestalt therapy, co-counselling and encounter group work (Shaffer, 1978).

A small number of those interviewed (n = 3) cited methods that involved altered states of consciousness, including meditation, trance work and neuro-linguistic programming (Bandler and Grinder, 1979). Others (n = 3) referred to games and simulations as examples of experiential learning methods. Only two mentioned the use of videos or TVs (as learning aids), and two referred to physical activities that involved active movement on the part of the learners. These examples were perhaps less diverse in their range than had been the definitions of experiential learning, and the methods cited by the interviewees were supported by the literature on experiential learning which tends to refer consistently to role play, structured activities and a range of 'therapeutic' activities (see for example Heron, 1973; Burnard, 1985).

Thus a broad range of definitions, but a narrow band of methods, emerged as a consistent trend. As we noted above, perhaps the fact that there is considerable agreement on the things that may be called experiential learning methods is more important, from a practical, educational point of view, than is the diversity of opinion over definitions of experiential learning. On the other hand, it may be that tutors and lecturers have taken on board the popular 'buzz words and phrases' in nurse education, without too much thought or consideration of how these new ideas may affect their teaching practice. If this latter scenario is at all accurate, the outlook for developing more caring and interpersonally skilled nurses in the future is far from promising.

What is not clear from this analysis is the degree to which the educators distinguish between educational activities and therapeutic activities. There may or may not be a contractual issue here: learners may come to an educational enterprise expecting to receive education. It would appear that some may receive 'therapy', in the form of the 'humanistic therapies' identified above or in terms of altered states of consciousness. The distinction between education and therapy clearly deserves greater clarification.

❏ **Comparison with other learning methods**

When asked for examples of learning methods other than experiential learning methods, the most frequently cited method was the lecture (n = 9). Other interviewees (n = 3) identified 'teacher-centred' methods: seminars, reading and watching videos. Again, this is in keeping with the literature on experiential and allied learning approaches, and particularly perhaps with the student-centred approach of the late humanistic educator and psychotherapist, Carl Rogers (1983), who stressed the need to avoid teacher-centred methods and lecturing in order to maximise learning from experience. The aim of this particular question was to identify a contrasting method with which the experiential learning approach could be compared.

❏ **Advantages of the experiential learning approach**

Interviewees were then asked to identify what they perceived as being the advantages of the experiential learning approach. Tables 10.3 and 10.4 illustrate the range of ideas generated in this area.

Table 10.3   Advantages of the experiential learning approach (n = 12)

Advantages	Frequency	Rank order
1. Useful for teaching interpersonal skills	5	= 1
2. Experiential learning increases self-awareness	5	= 1
3. 'Real/whole/active'	4	3
4. Light-hearted/fun	3	4
5. Lecturer enjoys using them	2	= 5
6. More relaxed than other methods	2	= 5
7. Useful for teaching practical nursing skills	2	= 5
8. Easier to use than other methods	1	8

The most frequently referred-to advantages of the approach were that they were useful for teaching interpersonal skills (n = 5) and that they increased self-awareness (n = 5). These points are reinforced by the literature on the topic (Kagan, 1985; Kagan *et al.*, 1986), although the concept of 'self-awareness' remains problematic and none of the interviewees offered a clear definition of what it was. Some of the interviewees (n = 4) referred to concepts such as 'real', 'whole' or 'active' as descriptors of the advantages of experiential learning. These are necessarily difficult to classify and perhaps to define. Only two of those interviewed saw experiential learning methods as advantageous in the teaching of practical nursing skills.

It is also notable that some (n = 3) saw them as being light-hearted or fun to use, while two saw them as being more relaxed in their approach than other methods, and one person identified them as being easier to use. 'Other' methods refers here to more traditional lecture- and teacher-centred approaches. It may be noted that in another study we carried out into preferred teaching and learning styles among student nurses and lecturers, we found that *lecturers* tended to prefer to use experiential learning approaches, while a majority of students were less clear about their preference for them (Burnard and Morrison, 1992).

Table 10.4   Disadvantages of the experiential learning approach (n = 12)

Disadvantages	Frequency	Rank order
1. Can be uncomfortable or threatening for the student	9	1
2. Not suitable for all topics on syllabus	5	2
3. Needs lots of planning	4	3
4. Time consuming	3	4

Interviewees were then asked about the disadvantages of the approach. Table 10.4 shows the sub-categories generated in this area. A majority of those interviewed (n = 9) acknowledged that learners undertaking experiential learning may find it uncomfortable or threatening. Many felt that this was because experiential learning was a more 'personal' approach to learning, as opposed to the more impersonal lecture method. As we have noted above, a limitation of this type of analysis is that it refers only to the overt content of the interview transcripts. It would be interesting to explore the latent content in this particular area. It may tentatively be hypothesised, for instance, that some of the discomfort and threat identified in this section may be projected discomfort and threat on the part of the educators. In other words, the perceived discomfort may have been an expression of the educator's own discomfort. This must remain conjecture, however, as the method of analysis does not allow for such a hypothesis to be tested.

However, the mention of threat and discomfort is again intriguing. Why would advocates of a particular approach, which incidentally is much more positive and encouraging in style than the traditional methods of learning, continue to use a mode of teaching which is disliked by the learners. Where, one asks, is the negotiated curriculum and the encouragement for the learner to have her say? These and similar questions may be answered in some part by the next stage of analysis.

Some (n = 5) suggested that a disadvantage may be that experiential learning was not suitable for all topics on the timetable, but it is interesting and perhaps paradoxical that others (n = 4) identified experiential learning (see above) as involving the whole of life experience. Furthermore, it is perhaps reasonable to expect that no one method will be suitable for learning or teaching all topics on a curriculum. The need to engage in lots of planning was identified as a disadvantage by four people, three found experiential learning time consuming and one was concerned with the issue of whether or not the learning gained from an experiential learning session could be carried over into the 'real' situation (the 'transfer of learning' problem). This issue has been discussed in more detail in the increasing literature on clinical teaching and ward-based training (Ogier, 1982; Fretwell, 1986).

❏ **Evaluating experiential learning**

The interviewees were then asked how they evaluated experiential learning. Table 10.5 outlines the sub-categories generated in this area. The most frequently cited method of evaluating experiential learning was to ask the learners to feed back their opinion of the usefulness or value of the experience at the end of an experiential learning session (n = 10). This method is frequently cited in the literature on experiential learning (Heron, 1973; Kilty, 1978, 1982; Burnard, 1985), although it perhaps allows only a very subjective, 'impressionistic' picture of learning to emerge. It also anticipates that learning can be evaluated very soon after the experience. It is arguable that other evaluation methods need to be used after some time has elapsed in order for full assimilation of the learning to take place (Clift and Imrie, 1981). Some of those interviewed (n = 5) said that they asked for written evaluation reports from their students, and a minority (n = 2) used repertory grid techniques (Fransella and Bannister, 1977). One said that she asked for reports from nurses working on the wards and used these as an indicator of the effectiveness or otherwise of experiential learning. Another reported that she observed the learners on the wards to evaluate them in a similar way. A number of the interviewees noted that evaluation of experiential learning was 'difficult' (n = 5). The subjective nature of experiential learning must continue to make the subject of evaluation an awkward one.

Table 10.5   Evaluation methods in experiential learning (n = 5)

Evaluation method	Frequency	Rank order
1. Verbal feedback from the group	10	1
2. Written reports from students	5	2
3. Repertory grid techniques	2	3
4. Reports from the wards	1	= 4
5. Observation	1	= 4

This study examined some perceptions of 12 nurse educators regarding experiential learning. Three particular issues are notable from the study:

• the diversity of opinion on how experiential learning is to be defined

- the fact that a high proportion of the interviewees noted that learners may be made to feel uncomfortable or threatened by the use of experiential learning activities, and
- the rather limited approach to evaluating experiential learning discussed by those interviewed.

While the small number of subjects in this study is a limitation, it is arguable that, given the diversity of opinion on what constitutes 'experiential learning', it is difficult to justify the 1982 syllabus's prescription of experiential learning as a preferred learning method. If experiential learning means different things to different people, there can be no guarantee that there will be any uniformity of interpretation of this syllabus. Clarifying the definition of experiential learning may have important consequences for training future nurse educators. If future tutors are to learn how to become experiential learning facilitators, it is important that there is some degree of agreement on what experiential learning is and what it is not.

It may be helpful, too, if further research were to be done to identify exactly what it is that some learners find uncomfortable about experiential learning and whether or not the tentative hypothesis about 'projected' discomfort, posed above, has any merit.

More work also needs to be carried out in the field of evaluating experiential learning. Given the subjective nature of the field and the centrality of individual experience, this would seem to be a particularly difficult area.

The study has offered an interesting 'glimpse' of how some nurse educators view experiential learning and is to be followed up by further work, particularly in the area of how learners view experiential learning. It will be interesting to note the degree of congruence or otherwise between educators' accounts of experiential learning and those offered by learners.

■ Summary

This chapter has explored the educational process known as experiential learning. It has argued that communication skills may best be learned through reference to nurses' own experience of life and work. The chapter has also described a variety of nurses' perceptions of experiential learning.

■ Conclusion

In this book, we have tried to highlight some of the things that make for an effective interpersonal relationship between nurses and patients. We noted, for example, the complexity of the concept we call 'caring'. We examined a range of studies into caring and indicated some ways in which you may want to think about your own caring relationships with patients, with their families and with colleagues. We also consider what it means to communicate with others. We identified various methods of classifying communication skills and suggested activities for helping you to become aware of your own interpersonal skills and honing them a little to make them more effective.

The important emphasis throughout the book has been that caring and communicating are inseparably linked. You cannot hope to communicate effectively if you do not care about the person on the receiving end. You only have to study some of the 'professional communicators' whom we find in shops and offices to establish this point. Next time you are being served by a person who has a glossy but 'empty' self-presentation, ponder on whether or not you feel to any degree *cared for* by that person. The point, then, is that you cannot simply adopt a set of behaviours that seem to make for effective communication. You must have the *affect* or feeling behind them that says 'I care about you'.

What counts most of all is how *you,* the reader, review and maintain your relationships with others. The point about all skills is that they need to be *practised.* To be an effective communicator, you need to practise your communication skills. Perhaps more difficult, however, is that you also need to *practise* caring. You need to practise giving something of your-self to others. Again, this is not easy. In the end, though, if we really want to be effective practitioners in nursing, we must find the means of combining both excellence in communication skills and a genuine desire to care for others.

References

Adams-Webber, J.R. 1979 *Personal Construct Theory.* John Wiley, Chichester.

Ajzen, I. 1988 *Attitudes, Personality and Behaviour.* Open University, Milton Keynes.

Altschul. A. 1972 *Patient-nurse Interaction.* Churchill-Livingstone, London.

Antonak, R.F. and Livneh, H. 1988 *The Measurement of Attitudes Toward People with Disabilities: Methods, psychometrics and scales.* Charles Thomas, Springfield, Illinois.

Argyle, M. 1985 *Anatomy of Relationships.* Penguin, Harmondsworth.

Ashworth, P.D. 1987 Adequacy of Description. The Validity of Qualitative Findings. Sheffield Papers in Education Management no. 67, Department of Education Management, Sheffield City Polytechnic.

Ashworth, P.D. and Morrison, P. 1989 Some ambiguities of the student's role in undergraduate nurse training. *Journal of Advanced Nursing,* **14:**1009–15.

Atkinson, R.I., Atkinson, R.C., Smith, E.E. and Bem, D.J. 1990 *Introduction to Psychology.* Harcourt Brace Jovanovitch, San Diego, California.

Audit Commission 1993 *What Seems to be the Matter: Communication between hospitals and patients.* HMSO, London.

Bandler, R. and Grinder, J. 1979 *Frogs into Princes: Neuro linguistic programming.* Real People Press, Moab, Utah.

Bannister, D. and Fransella, F. 1986 *Inquiring Man,* 3rd edn. Croom Helm, London.

Bannister, D. and Mair, J.M.M. 1968 *The Evaluation of Personal Constructs.* Academic Press, London.

Baron, R.A. 1985 Reducing organisational conflict: the role of attributions. *Journal of Applied Psychology,* **70:**434–41.

Baron, R.A. and Byrne, D. 1987 *Social Psychology: Understanding human interation,* 5th edn. Allyn and Bacon, Boston.

Beail, N. 1985 *Repertory Grid Technique and Personal Constructs.* Croom Helm, London.

Bem, D.J. 1972 Self-perception theory. In L. Berkowitz (ed.) *Advances in Experimental Social Psychology,* vol. 6. Academic Press, New York.

Ben-Sira, Z. 1976 The function of the professional's affective behaviour in client satisfaction: a revised approach to social interaction theory. *Journal of Health and Social Behaviour,* **17:**3–11.

Ben-Sira, Z. 1980 Affective and instrumental components in the physician–patient relationship: an additional dimension of interaction theory. *Journal of Health and Social Behaviour,* **21:**170–80.

Ben-Sira, Z. 1983 The structure of a hospital's image. *Medical Care,* **21**(10):943–54.

Bendall, E. 1977 The future of British nurse education. *Journal of Advanced Nursing*, **2**:171–81.

Blake, R.R. and Mouton, J.S. 1976 *Consultation*. Addison Wesley, New York.

Bogdan, R.C. and Biklen, S.K. 1982 *Qualitative Research for Education: An introduction to theory and methods*. Alleyn and Bacon, Toronto.

Bond, M. and Kilty, J. 1983 *Practical Methods of Dealing With Stress*. HPRP, University of Surrey, Guildford.

Boore, J. 1978 *A Prescription for Recovery*. RCN, London.

Borg, I. and Lingoes, J. 1987 *Multidimensional Similarity Structure Analysis*. Springer-Verlag, New York.

Brearley, S. 1990 *Patient Participation: The literature*. RCN Research Series. Scutari Press, Harrow.

Breckler, S.J. 1984 Empirical validation of affect, behaviour and cognition as distinct components of attitude. *Journal of Personality and Social Psychology*, **47**:1191–205.

Brookfield, S. 1987 *Developing Critical Thinkers: Challenging adults to explore alternative ways of thinking and acting*. Open University Press, Milton Keynes.

Brown, L. 1982 Behaviours of nurses perceived by hospitalized patients as indicators of care, *Dissertation Abstracts International*, **42**(11):4361-b.

Buber, M. 1958 *I and Thou*. New York, Scribener.

Buber, M. 1966 *The Knowledge of Man: A philosophy of the interhuman*, M. Freidman (ed.), R.G. Smith (trans.). Harper & Row, New York.

Burnard, P. 1983 Through experience and from experience. *Nursing Times*, **156**(9):29–34.

Burnard, P. 1984 A Critical Review of the Concept of Experiential Learning with Special Reference to the Training of Student Psychiatric Nurses. MSc Dissertation, University of Surrey, Guildford.

Burnard, P. 1984 Counselling the nurses. *Nursing Mirror*, **159**(40):30–1.

Burnard, P. 1985 *Learning Human Skills: A guide for nurses*. Heinemann, London.

Burnard, P. 1989a *Teaching Interpersonal Skills: A handbook of experiential learning for health professionals*. Chapman & Hall, London.

Burnard, P. 1989b *Counselling Skills for Health Professionals*. Chapman & Hall, London.

Burnard, P. 1990 *Learning Human Skills*, 2nd edn. Butterworth-Heinemann, Oxford.

Burnard, P. 1994 *Counselling Skills for Health Professionals*, 2nd edn. Chapman & Hall, London.

Burnard, P. and Morrison, P. 1988 Nurses' perceptions of their interpersonal skills: a descriptive study using Six Category Intervention Analysis. *Nurse Education Today*, **8**:266–72.

Burnard, P. and Morrison, P. 1991 Nurses' interpersonal skills: a study of nurses' perceptions. *Nurse Education Today*, **11**: 24–9.

Burnard, P. and Morrison, P. 1992 Students' and lecturers' preferred teaching strategies. *International Journal of Nursing Studies*, **29**(4):345–53.

Campbell, A.V. 1984a *Paid to Care?* SPCK, London.

Campbell, A.V. 1984b *Moderated Love: A theology of professional care*. SPCK, London.

Carney, T.F. 1972 *Content Analysis*. University of Manitoba Press, Manitoba, Canada.

Carper, B.A. 1979 The ethics of caring. *Advances in Nursing Science*, **1**(3):11–19.

Chapman, C.M. 1983 The paradox of nursing. *Journal of Advanced Nursing,* **8**:269–72.

Choppin, R.G. 1983 *The Role of the Ward Sister: a review of the British research literature since 1967.* Project Paper no. 33. Kings Fund Centre, London.

Clifford, C. 1995 Caring: fitting the concept to nursing practice. *Journal of Clinical Nursing,* **4**:37–41.

Clift, J.C. and Imrie, B.W. 1981 *Assessing Students: Appraising students.* Croom Helm, London.

Cohen, J.S. and Struening, E.L. 1959 Factors underlying opinions about mental illness in the personnel in a large mental hospital. *American Psychologist,* **14**:339.

Cohen, J.S. and Struening, E.L. 1960 Attitudes towards the mentally ill of psychiatric hospital personnel as a function of occupation, education, age and sex. *American Psychologist,* **15**:417.

Cohen, S. 1981 Patient education: a review of the literature. *Journal of Advanced Nursing,* **6**:11–18.

Coke, J.S., Batson, C.D. and McDavis, K. 1978 Empathic mediation of helping: a two stage model. *Journal of Personality and Social Psychology,* **36**:752–66.

Coleman, J.S. 1958 Relational analysis: the study of social organisations with survey methods. *Human Organisation,* **17**:28–36.

Cook, S.W. and Selltiz, C. 1973 A multiple indicator approach to attitude measurement. In N. Warren and M. Jahoda (eds) *Attitudes,* 2nd edn. Penguin, Harmondsworth.

Cope, D.E. 1981 *Organisation Development and Action Research in Hospitals.* Gower, London.

Costigan, J., Humphrey, J. and Murphy, C. 1987 Attempted suicide: a personal construct psychology exploration. *Australian Journal of Advanced Nursing,* **4**(2):39–50.

Cowen, E.L. 1982 Help is where you find it. *American Psychologist,* **37**(4):385–95.

Cox, M. 1978 *Structuring the Therapuetic Process.* Pergamon Press, London.

Crowne, D.P. and Marlowe, D. 1964 *The Approval Motive.* John Wiley, New York.

Davis, B.D. 1983 A Repertory Grid Study of Formal and Informal Aspects of Student Nurse Training. PhD Thesis, London University, School of Economics.

Devine, E.C. and Cook, T.D. 1983 A meta-analytical analysis of effects of psychoeducational interventions on length of postsurgical hospital stay. *Nursing Research,* **32**(5):267–74.

DiMatteo, M.R. and DiNicola, D.D. 1982 *Achieving Patient Compliance: The psychology of the medical practitioner's role.* Pergamon Press, New York.

Drew, N. 1986 Exclusion and confirmation: a phenomenology of patients' experiences with care givers. *Image – Journal of Nursing Scholarship,* **18**(2): 39–43.

Dryden, W. 1985 Teaching counselling skills to non-psychologists. *British Journal of Medical Psychology,* **58**:217–22.

Duck, S.W. 1973 *Personal Relationships and Personal Constructs.* John Wiley, Chichester.

Easterby-Smith, M. 1981 The design, analysis and interpretation of repertory grids. In M.L.G. Shaw (ed.) *Recent Advances in Personal Construct Technology.* Academic Press, London.

Egan, G. 1986 *The Skilled Helper.* Brooks Cole, Monterey, California.

Egbert L.D., Battit, G.E., Welch C.E. and Bartlett, M.K. 1964 Reduction of postoperative pain by encouragement and instruction of patients. *New England Journal of Medicine*, **270**(16):825–7.

Eisenberg-Berg, N. and Geisheker, E. 1979 Content of preachings and power of the model/preacher: the effect on children's generosity. *Developmental Psychology*, **15**:168–75.

ENB 1982 *Syllabus of Training: Professional Register – Part 3 (Registered Mental Nurse)*. English and Welsh National Boards for Nursing Midwifery and Health Visiting, London.

ENB 1987 *Managing Change in Nurse Education. Pack One: Preparing for Change*. English National Board with Learning Materials Design, Sheffield.

Epting, F. 1984 *Personal Construct Counselling and Psychotherapy*. John Wiley, Chichester.

Fazio, R.H. 1986 How do attitudes guide behaviour? In R.M. Sorrentino and E.M. Higgins (eds) *The Handbook of Motivation and Cognition: Foundations of social behaviour*. Guildford, New York.

Fazio, R.H., Chen, J., McDonel, E.C. and Sherman, S.J. 1982 Attitude accessibility, attitude-behaviour consistency and the strength of the object-evaluation association. *Journal of Experimental Social Psychology*, **18**:339–57.

Ferguson, B.F. 1979 Preparing young children for hospitalization: a comparison of two methods. *Pediatrics*, **64**(5):656–64.

Festinger, L. 1957 *A Theory of Cognitive Dissonance*. Row, Peterson, New York.

Field, P.A. and Morse, J.M. 1985 *Nursing Research: The application of qualitative approaches*. Croom Helm, London.

Fielding, R.G. and Llewelyn, S.P. 1987 Communication training in nursing may damage your health and enthusiasm: some warnings. *Journal of Advanced Nursing*, **12**:281–90.

Fink, A. and Kosecoff, J. 1985 *How To Conduct Surveys*. Sage, Beverely Hills, California.

Fisher, W.F. 1963 Sharing in pre-school children as a function of amount and type of reinforcement. *Genetic Psychology Monographs*, **68**:215–45.

Ford, M.B. 1981 Nurse Professionals and the Caring Process. Dissertation for EdD, University of Northern Colorado.

Forgas, J.P. 1979 Multidimensional scaling: a discovery method in social psychology. In G.P. Ginsburg (ed.) *Emerging Strategies in Social Psychological research*. John Wiley, Chichester.

Forrest, D. 1989 The experience of caring. *Journal of Advanced Nursing*, **14**:815–23.

Fransella, F. and Bannister, D. 1977 *A Manual for Repertory Grid Technique*. Academic Press, London.

Fretwell, J. 1982 *Ward Teaching and Learning*. RCN, London.

Fretwell, J. 1986 *Freedom to Change*. RCN, London.

Fry, S.T. 1988 The ethics of caring: can it survive in nursing? *Nursing Outlook*, **36**(1):48.

Giorgi, A. 1970 *Psychology as a Human Science: A phenomenologically based approach*. Harper & Row, New York.

Goffman, E. 1961 *Asylums*. Doubleday, Garden City, New York.

Goodman, C. 1986 Research on the informal carer: a selected literature review. *Journal of Advanced Nursing*, **11**:705–12.

Griffin, A.P. 1980 Philosophy and nursing. *Journal of Advanced Nursing*, **5**:261–72.

Griffin, A.P. 1983 A philosophical analysis of caring in nursing. *Journal of Advanced Nursing*, **8**:289–95.

Hall, J.N. 1990 Towards a psychology of caring. *British Journal of Clinical Psychology*, **29**:129–44.

Hall, L. 1966 Another view of nursing care and quality. In K. Straub and K. Parker (eds) *Continuity of Patient Care: The role of nursing*. Catholic University Press, Washington, DC.

Hammond, G.H. 1983 A clutch of concepts. *Nursing Mirror*, 11 May, 34–5.

Harris, B. and Harvey, J.H. 1981 Attribution theory: from phenomenal causality to the intuitive social scientist and beyond. In C. Antaki (ed.) *The Psychology of Ordinary Explanations of Social Behaviour*. Academic Press, London.

Harris, S., Mussen, P. and Rutherford, E. 1976 Some cognitive, behavioural and personality correlates of maturity and moral judgement. *Journal of Genetic Psychology*, **128**:123–35.

Hayward, J. 1975 *Information: A prescription against pain*. RCN, London.

Heider, F. 1958 *The Psychology of Interpersonal Relations*. John Wiley, New York.

Henneman, L. 1984 Systems run best downhill: facilitating change in organisations. In S. Simpson, P. Higson, R. Holland, J. McBrien, J. Williams, and L. Henneman (eds) *Facing the Challenge*. BABP Publications, Rossendale, Lancashire.

Henry, O.M.M. 1975 Nurse behaviours perceived by patients as indicators of caring. *Dissertation Abstracts International*, 75–16, 299, 652-b.

Heron, J. 1973 *Experiential Training Techniques*. HPRP, University of Surrey, Guildford.

Heron, J. 1975 *Six Category Intervention Analysis*. HPRP, University of Surrey, Guildford.

Heron, J. 1977a *Behaviour Analysis in Education and Training*. HPRP, University of Surrey, Guildford.

Heron, J. 1977b *Catharsis in Human Development*. HPRP, University of Surrey, Guildford.

Heron, J. 1986 *Six Category Intervention Analysis*, 2nd edn. HPRP, University of Surrey, Guildford.

Heron, J. 1989 *Six Category Intervention Analysis*, 3rd edn. HPRP, University of Surrey, Guildford.

Heron, J. 1990 *Helping the Client*. Sage, London.

Heyman, R., Shaw, M.P. and Harding, J. 1983 A personal construct theory approach to the socialisation of nursing trainees in two British general hospitals. *Journal of Advanced Nursing*, **8**:59–67.

Hirschfeld, M. 1983 Home care versus institutionalization: family caregiving and senile brain disease. *International Journal of Nursing Studies*, **20**(1):23–32.

Holmes, C.A. (1990) Alternatives to natural science foundations for nursing. *International Journal of Nursing Studies*, **27**(3):187–98.

Holtzworth-Munroe, A. and Jacobson, N.S. 1985 Causal attributions of married couples: when do they search for causes? What do they conclude when they do? *Journal of Personality and Social Psychology*, **48**:1398–412.

Homans, G.C. 1961 *Social Behaviour in its Elementary Forms*. Harcourt Brace, New York.

Honess, T. 1985 Repertory grids and the psychological case study. In N. Beail (ed.) *Repertory Grid Technique and Personal Constructs*. Croom Helm, London.

Honey, P. 1979 The repertory grid in action. *Industrial and Commercial Training*, **11**(9):358–69.

Human Potential Research Project, 1987 *Prospectus of Workshops and Short Courses.* HPRP, University of Surrey, Guildford.

Hyde, A. 1976 The phenomenon of caring. *Nursing Research Report,* **11**(3):2, 19.

Jacobson, S.F. and McGrath, H.M. 1983 *Nurses under Stress.* John Wiley, New York.

Jeffrey, R. (1979) Normal rubbish: deviant patients in casualty departments. *Sociology of Health and Illness,* **1**(1):90–107.

Johnson, M. and Jones, M.L. 1979 Evaluating the care of post-surgical patients in the community hospital. In D.J. Oborne, M.M. Gruneberg and J.R. Eiser (eds) *Research in Psychology and Medicine,* vol. 2. Academic Press, London.

Jones, E.E. and Davis, K.E. 1965 From acts to dispositions: the attribution process in person perception. In L. Berkowitz (ed.) *Advances in Experimental Social Psychology.* vol. 2. Academic Press, New York.

Jourard, S. 1964 *The Transparent Self.* Van Nostrand, New York.

Jourard, S. 1971 *Self-Disclosure: An experimental analysis of the transparent self.* John Wiley, New York.

Kagan, C. (ed.) 1985 *Interpersonal Skills in Nursing: Research and applications.* Croom Helm, London.

Kagan, C., Evans, J. and Kay, B. 1986 *A Manual of Interpersonal Skills for Nurses: An experiential approach.* Harper & Row, London.

Kanekar, S., Pinto, N.J.P. and Mazumdar, D. 1985 Causal and moral responsibility of victims of rape and robbery. *Journal of Applied Social Psychology,* **15**:622–37.

Kelley, H.H. 1972 Attributions in social interaction. In E.E. Jones *et al.* (eds) *Attribution: Perceiving the causes of behaviour.* General Learning Press, Morristown, New Jersey.

Kelly, G.A. 1955 *The Psychology of Personal Constructs,* vols 1 and 2. Norton, New York.

Kelly, G.A. 1963 *A Theory of Personality: The psychology of personal constructs.* Norton, New York.

Kelly, G.A. 1969 The autobiography of a theory. In B.A. Maher (ed.) *Clinical Psychology and Personality, Selected Papers of George Kelly.* John Wiley, New York.

Kelly, M.P. and May, P. 1982 Good and bad patients: a review of the literature and a theoretical critique. *Journal of Advanced Nursing,* **7**:147–56.

Kenny, C. and Canter, D. 1979 Patient experience and ward design. In D.J. Oborne, M.M. Gruneberg and J.R. Eiser (eds) *Research in Psychology and Medicine,* vol. 2. Academic Press, London.

Kestenbaum, V. (ed.) 1982a *The Humanity of the Ill: Phenomenological perspectives.* University of Tenessee Press, Knoxville.

Kestenbaum, V. 1982b Introduction: the experience of illness. In V. Kestenbaum (ed.) *The Humanity of the Ill: Phenomenological perspectives.* University of Tennessee Press, Knoxville.

Kilty, J. 1978 *Self and Peer Assesment.* HPRP, University of Surrey, Guildford.

Kilty, J. 1982 *Experiential Learning.* HPRP, University of Surrey, Guildford.

Kitson, A.L. 1987 A comparative analysis of lay-caring and professional (nursing) caring relationships. *International Journal of Nursing Studies,* **2**(2):155–65.

Knight, M. and Field, D. 1981 A silent conspiracy: coping with dying cancer patients on an acute surgical ward. *Journal of Advanced Nursing,* **6**:212–29.

Knowles, M.S. 1986 *Using Learning Contracts.* Jossey Bass, San Francisco, California.

Krebs, D. 1978 A cognitive-development approach to altruism. In L. Wispe (ed.) *Altruism, Sympathy and Helping: Psychological and sociological principles.* New York, Academic Press.

Kruskal, J.B. and Wish, M. 1978 *Multidimensional Scaling.* Sage, London.

Kyle, T.V. 1995 The concept of caring: a review of the literature. *Journal of Advanced Nursing,* **21**:506–14.

Lalljee, M. 1981 Attribution theory and the analysis of explanations. In C. Antaki (ed.) *The Psychology of Ordinary Explanations of Social Behaviour.* Academic Press, London.

Landfield, A.W. 1971 *Personal Construct Systems in Psychotherapy.* Rand McNally, Chicago.

Larson, P.J. 1984 Important nurse caring behaviours perceived by patients with cancer. *Oncology Nursing Forum,* **11**(6):46–50.

Lecky, P. 1961 *Self-Consistency: A theory of personality.* Shoe String Press, Hamden, Connecticut.

Leigh, H. and Reiser, M.F. 1980 *The Patient: Biological, psychological, and social dimensions of medical practice.* Plenum Press, New York.

Leininger, M.M. 1977 The phenomenon of caring, Part 5. *Nursing Research Report,* **12**(1):2, 14.

Leininger, M.M. 1981a The phenomenon of caring: importance, research questions and theoretical considerations. In M.M. Leininger (ed.) *Caring: An essential human need.* Charles B. Slack, New Jersey.

Leininger, M.M. 1981b Some philosophical, historical, and taxonomic aspects of nursing and caring in American culture. In M.M. Leininger (ed.) *Caring: An essential human need.* Charles B. Slack, New Jersey.

Leino-Kilpi, H., Iire, L., Suominen, T., Vuorenheimo, J. and Valimaki, M. 1993 Client and information: a literature review. *Journal of Clinical Nursing,* **2**:331–40.

Lelean, S.R. 1973 *Ready for Report Nurse? A Study in Nursing Communication in Hospital Wards.* RCN, London.

Ley, P. 1988 *Communicating with Patients: Improving communication, satisfaction and compliance.* Chapman & Hall, London.

Lifshitz, M. 1974 Quality professionals: does training make a difference? A personal construct theory study of the issue. *British Journal of Social and Clinical Psychology,* **13**:183–9.

Lingoes, J.C. 1973 *The Guttman–Lingoes Nonmetric Program Series.* Mathesis Press, Ann Arbor, Michigan.

Livingston, M. and Livingston, H. 1984 Emotional distress in nurses at work. *British Journal of Medical Psychology,* **57**:291–4.

Llewelyn, S.P. 1984 The cost of giving: emotional growth and emotional stress. In S. Skevington (ed.) *Understanding Nurses.* John Wiley, Chichester.

Llewelyn, S.P. 1989 Caring: the cost to nurses and relatives. In A. Broome (ed.) *Health Psychology: Processes and applications.* Chapman & Hall, London.

Lorber, J. 1975 Good patients and problem patients: conformity and deviance in a general hospital. *Journal of Health and Social Behaviour,* **16**(2):213–25.

McFarlane, J. 1976 A charter for caring. *Journal of Advanced Nursing,* **1**:187–96.

Macleod Clark, J. and Faulkner, A. 1987 Communication skills teaching in nurse education. In B. Davis (ed.) *Nursing Education: Research and Developments.* Croom Helm, London.

Marshall, J. 1980 *White Collar and Professional Stress.* John Wiley, Chichester.

Marson, S.N. 1982 Ward sister – teacher or facilitator? An investigation into the behavioural characteristics of effective ward teachers. *Journal of Advanced Nursing*, 7:347–57.

May, R. 1983 *The Discovery of Being*. Norton, New York.

Mayeroff, M. 1972 *On Caring*. Harper & Row, London.

Melia, K. 1987 *Learning and Working: The occupational socialisation of nurses*. Tavistock, London.

Menzies, I.E.P. 1970 *The Functioning of Social Systems as a Defence Against Anxiety*. Centre for Applied Social Research, Tavistock Institute of Human Relations, London.

Meyer, J.P. and Mulherin, A. 1980 From attribution to helping: an analysis of the mediating effects of affect and expectancy. *Journal of Personality and Social Psychology*, **39**:201–10.

Miles, M.B. and Huberman, A.M. 1994 *Qualitative Data Analysis*. Sage, London.

Moores, B. and Grant, G.W.B. 1977 The 'avoidance' syndrome in hospitals for the mentally handicapped. *International Journal of Nursing Studies*, **1**:91–5.

Morris, D. 1978 *Manwatching*. Triad, St Albans.

Morrison, P. 1989a Nursing and caring: a personal construct theory study of some nurses' self-perceptions. *Journal of Advanced Nursing*, **14**:421–6.

Morrison, P. 1989b The caring attitude: nurses' self-perceptions. *Nursing Times*, **85**(4):56.

Morrison, P. 1991 The Meaning of Caring Interpersonal Relationships in Nursing. PhD Thesis. Sheffield Hallam University, Sheffield.

Morrison, P. 1992 *Professional Caring in Practice. A psychological analysis*. Avebury, Aldershot.

Morrison, P. 1994 *Understanding Patients*. Baillière Tindall, London.

Morrison, P. and Bauer, I. 1993 A clinical application of the multiple sorting technique. *International Journal of Nursing Studies*, **30**(6):511–18.

Morrison, P. and Burnard, P. 1989 Students' and trained nurses' perceptions of their own interpersonal skills: a report and comparison. *Journal of Advanced Nursing*, **14**:321–9.

Morrison, P., Burnard, P. and Hackett, P. 1991 A smallest space analysis of nurses' perceptions of their interpersonal skills. *Counselling Psychology Quarterly*, **4**(2/3):115–21.

Myerscough, P.R. 1989 *Talking with Patients: A basic clinical skill*. Oxford Medical Publications, Oxford.

Neimeyer, R.A., Fontana, D.J. and Gold, K. 1984 A manual for content analysis of death constructs. In F.R. Epting and R.A. Neimeyer (eds) *Personal Meanings of Death*. McGraw-Hill, London.

Nelson-Jones, R. 1982 *The Theory and Practice of Counselling Psychology*. Holt, Rinehart and Winston, London.

Nelson-Jones, R. 1995 *The Theory and Practice of Counselling*. Cassell, London.

Nelson-Jones, R. and Patterson, C.H. Measuring client-centred attitudes. *British Journal of Guidance and Counselling*, **3**(2):228–36.

New, P.K., Nite, G. and Callahan, J. 1959 Too many nurses may be worse than too few. *Modern Hospital*, **4**:104–7.

Nichols, K.A. 1985 Psychological care by nurses, paramedical and medical staff: essential developments for the general hospitals. *British Journal of Medical Psychology*, **58**:231–40.

Nicolas, B. and Gooderham, D. 1982 Mental Nursing. 1: Devising and implementing new syllabuses for mental and mental handicap nurse training. *Nursing Times*, 17 March, Quest 2 and 3, 76–9.

Nolan, M.R. and Grant, G. 1989 Addressing the needs of informal carers: a neglected area of nursing practice. *Journal of Advanced Nursing*, 14:950–61.

Nyatanga, L. 1989 The Q-Sort theory and technique. *Nurse Education Today*, 9:347–50.

Ogier, M. 1982 *An Ideal Sister*. RCN, London.

Ogier, M. 1984 How do ward sisters influence learning by nurses in the wards. In S. Skevington (ed.) *Understanding Nurses*. John Wiley, Chichester.

Omery, A. 1983 Phenomenology: a method for nursing research. *Advances in Nursing Science*, 5(2):49–63.

Orton, H.D. 1981 *Ward Learning Climate: A study of the role of the ward sister in relation to student nurse learning on the ward*. RCN, London.

Partridge, K.B. 1978 Nursing values in a changing society. *Nursing Outlook*, June, 356–60.

Pearce, P., Amato, P.R. and Smithson, M. 1983 Introduction and plan of the book. In M. Smithson, P.R. Amato and P. Pearce (eds) *Dimensions of Helping Behaviour*. Pergamon Press, Oxford.

Pembrey, S. 1987 Support your ward sister. *Nursing Times*, 30(39):27–9.

Peterson, M. 1988 The norms and values held by three groups of nurses concerning psychosocial nursing practice. *International Journal of Nursing Studies*, 25(2):85–103.

Pfeiffer J.W. and Jones, J.E. 1974 and ongoing. *A Handbook of Structured Experiences for Human Relations Training*. University Associates, La Jolla, California.

Pines, A.M., Aronson, E. and Kafry, D. 1981 *Burnout: From tedium to personal growth*. Free Press, Glencoe, New York.

Pinkus, L. and Dare, D. 1975 *Secrets in the Family*. Faber, London.

Pollock, L.C. 1987 Community Psychiatric Nursing Explained: An Analysis of the Views of Patients, Carers and Nurses. PhD Thesis, University of Edinburgh.

Posner, T.N. 1994 Technological control and healing: an uneasy combination? *Australian and New Zealand Journal of Mental Health Nursing*, 3(2):63–71.

Pratt, R. 1980 A time to every purpose.... *Australian Nurses' Journal*, 10(3):50–3, 56.

Pryor, J.B., Gibbons, F.X., Wicklund, R.A., Fazio, R.H. and Hood, R. 1977 Self-focused attention and self-report validity. *Journal of Personality*, 45:514–27.

Radsma, J. 1994 Caring and nursing: a dilemma. *Journal of Advanced Nursing*, 20:444–9.

Rajecki, D.W. 1982 *Attitudes: Themes and advances*. Sinauer, Sunderland, Massachusetts.

Raps, C.S., Peterson C., Jonas, M. and Seligman, M.E.P. 1982 Patient behaviour in hospitals: helplessness, reactance, or both? *Journal of Personality and Social Psychology*, 42(6):1036–41.

Rawlinson, J. W. 1995 Some reflections on the use of Repertory Grid Technique in studies of nurses and social workers. *Journal of Advanced Nursing*, 21:334–9.

Ray, M.A. 1981a A philosophical analysis of caring within nursing. In M.M. Leininger (ed.) *Caring: An essential human need*. Charles B. Slack, New Jersey.

Ray, M.A. 1981b A study of caring within an institutional culture. *Dissertation Abstracts International*, 42(6):2310-b.

Reason, P. and Rowan, J. 1981 *Human Inquiry: A sourcebook of new paradigm research*. John Wiley, Chichester.

Reiser, S. 1978 *Medicine and the Reign of Technology*. Cambridge University Press, Cambridge.

Rempusheski, V.F., Chamberlain, S.L., Picard, H.B., Ruzanski, J. and Collier, M. 1988 Expected and received care: patient perceptions. *Nursing Administration Quarterly*, **12**(3):42–50.

Robinson, J., Stilwell, J., Hawley, C. and Hempsted, N. 1989 *The Role of the Support Worker in the Ward Health Care Team*. Nursing Policy Studies Centre and Health Service Research Unit, University of Warwick.

Rogers, C.R. 1951 *Client-centred Therapy*. Constable, London.

Rogers, C.R. 1967 *On Becoming a Person: A therapist's view of psychotherapy*. Constable, London.

Rogers, C.R. 1983 *Freedom to Learn for the Eighties:* Merrill, Columbus, Ohio.

Roghmann, K.J., Hengst, A. and Zastowny, T.R. 1979 Satisfaction with medical care: its measurement and relation to utilisation. *Medical Care*, **17**:461.

Rowan, J. 1988 *Ordinary Ecstasy: Humanistic psychology in action*, 2nd edn. Routledge, London.

Rushton, J.P. 1980 *Altruism, Socialization and Society*. Prentice Hall, Englewood Cliffs, New Jersey.

Sarason, S.B. 1985 *Caring and Compassion in Clinical Practice*. Jossey-Bass, London.

Sartre, J.-P. 1952 *Existentialism and Humanism*. Methuen, London.

Sathe, V. 1983 Implications of corporate culture: a manager's guide to action. *Organisational Dynamics,* **12**:5–23.

Schein, E.H. 1984 Coming to a new awareness of organizational culture. *Sloan Management Review*, Winter, 3–16.

Schiffman, S.S., Reynolds, M.L. and Young, F.W. 1981 *Introduction to Multidimensional Scaling: Theory, methods and applications*. Academic Press, London.

Schwartz, S.H. 1977 Normative influences on altruism. In L. Berkowitz (ed.) *Advances in Experimental Social Psychology*, vol. 10. New York, Academic Press.

Selection Research Limited 1987 *A Selection Interview for Nurses in the National Health Service*. Selection Research, Surrey.

Shaffer, J.B.P. 1978 *Humanistic Psychology*. Prentice Hall, Englewood Cliffs, New Jersey.

Shapira, Z. 1976 A facet analysis of leadership styles. *Journal of Applied Psychology*, **61**:136–9.

Sivacek, J. and Crano, W.D. 1982 Vested interest as a moderator of attitude-behaviour consistency. *Journal of Personality and Social Psychology*, **43**:210–21.

Skipper, J.K. and Leonard, R.C. 1968 Children, stress, and hospitalisation: a field experiment. *Journal of Health and Social Behaviour*, **9**:275–87.

Smith, H.W. 1981 *Strategies of Social Research: The methodological imagination*, 2nd edn. Prentice Hall, Englewood Cliffs, New Jersey.

Smithson, M., Amato, P.R. and Pearce, P. (eds) 1983 *Dimensions of Helping Behaviour*. Pergamon Press, Oxford.

Sofer, C. 1955 Reactions to administrative change. *Human Relations*, **8**:291–316.

Spinelli, E. 1989 *The Interpreted World: An introduction to phenomenological psychology*. Sage, London.

Stewart, V. and Stewart, A. 1981 *Business Applications of Repertory Grid*. McGraw-Hill, London.

Stockwell, F. 1972 *The Unpopular Patient*. RCN, London.

Swanson-Kauffman, K. and Schonwald, E. 1988 Phenomenology. In B. Sarter (ed.) *Paths to Knowledge: Innovative research methods for nursing*. National League for Nursing, New York.

Taylor, D.S. 1990 Making the most of your matrices: hermenutics, statistics and the repertory grid. *International Journal of Personal Construct Psychology*, **3**:105–19.

Taylor, S.E. 1979 Hospital patient behaviour: reactance, helplessness, or control? *Journal of Social Issues*, **35**:156–84.

Taylor, S.J. and Bogdan, R. 1984 *Introduction to Qualitative Research Methods: The search for meanings*. John Wiley, Chichester.

Valle, R.S., King, M. and Halling, S. 1989 An introduction to existential-phenomenological thought in psychology. In R.S. Valle and S. Halling (eds) *Existential-phenomenological Perspectives in Psychology: Exploring the breadth of human experience*. Plenum Press, New York.

Wallis, D. 1987 Satisfaction, stress, and performance: issues for occupational psychology in the 'caring' professions. *Work and Stress*, **1**(2):113–28.

Waterworth, S. and Luker, K.A. 1990 Reluctant collaborators: do patients want to be involved in decisions concerning care? *Journal of Advanced Nursing*, **15**:971–6.

Watkins, J. 1978 *The Therapeutic Self*. Human Science Press, New York.

Watson, J. 1979 *Nursing: The philosophy and science of caring*. Little, Brown, Boston.

Watson, J. 1985 *Nursing: Human science and human care: A theory of nursing*. Appleton-Century-Crofts, New York.

Weil, S.W. and McGill, I. 1989 *Making Sense of Experiential Learning: Diversity in theory and practice*. Open University Press, Milton Keynes.

Weiner, B. 1980 A cognitive (attribution)-emotion-action model of motivated behaviour: an analysis of judgements of help-giving. *Journal of Personality and Social Psychology*, **39**:186–200.

Wicker, A.W. 1969 Attitudes versus actions: the relationship of verbal and overt behavioural responses to attitude objects. *Journal of Social Issues*, **25**:41–78.

Wilkinson, D. 1982 The effects of brief psychiatric training on the attitudes of general nursing students to psychiatric patients. *Journal of Advanced Nursing*, **7**:239–53.

Wilson, A.T.M. 1950 Hospital nursing auxiliaries. *Human Relations*, **3**(1):89–105.

Wilson, T.D. and Linville, P.W. 1982 Improving the academic performance of college freshmen: attribution theory revisited. *Journal of Personality and Social Psychology*, **42**:367–76.

Wilson-Barnett, J. 1984 Interventions to alleviate patient's stress: a review. *Journal of Psychosomatic Research*, **28**:63–72.

Further reading

Adams, J. (ed.) 1980 *Understanding and Managing Stress*. University Associates, San Diego, California.

Alberti, R.E. and Emmons, M.L. 1982 *Your Perfect Right: A guide*. Open Software Library, Wigan.

Alexander, F.M. 1969 *Resurrection of the Body*. University Books, New York.

Allan, D.M.E., Grosswald, S.J. and Means, R.P. 1984 Facilitating self-directed learning. In J.S. Green, S.J. Grosswald, E. Suter and D.B. Walthall (eds) *Continuing Education for the Health Professions: Developing, managing and evaluating programs for maximum impact on patient care*. Jossey Bass, San Francisco, California.

Allen, J. 1989 *How to Develop Your Personal Management Skills*. Kogan Page, London.

Alvino, D. 1986 A caring concept: providing information to make decisions. *Topics in Clinical Nursing*, **8**(2):70–6.

Anderson, H. and Gerrard, B. 1984 A comprehensive interpersonal skills program for nurses. *Journal of Nursing Education*, **23**(8):353–5.

Archer, R.L., Diaz-Loving, R., Gollwitzer, P.M., Davis, M.H. and Foushee, H.C. 1981 The role of dispositional empathy and social evaluation in the empathic mediation of helping. *Journal of Personality and Social Psychology*, **40**:786–96.

Argyris, C. 1982 *Reasoning, Learning and Action*. Jossey Bass, San Francisco.

Argyris, C. and Schon, D. 1974 *Theory in Practice: Increasing professional effectiveness*. Jossey Bass, San Francisco.

Argyris, C. and Schon, D. 1978 *Organisational Learning*. Addison Wesley, Reading, Massachusetts.

Astbury, C. 1988 *Stress in Theatre Nurses*. RCN, London.

Atwood, A.H. 1979 The mentor in clinical practice. *Nursing Outlook*, **27**:714–17.

Bailey, R. 1985 *Coping With Stress in Caring*. Blackwell, Oxford.

Bailey, R. and Clarke, M. 1989 *Stress and Coping in Nursing*. Chapman & Hall, London.

Baird, R.M. 1976 Existentialism, death and caring. *Journal of Religion and Health*, **15**(2):108–15.

Bannister, D. and Fransella, F. 1980 *Inquiring Man*, 2nd edn. Penguin, Harmondsworth.

Barker, P. 1989 Reflections on the philosophy of caring in mental health. *International Journal of Nursing Studies*, **26**(2):131–41.

Barrett-Lennard, G.T. 1981 The empathy cycle: refinement of a nuclear concept. *Journal of Counselling Psychology*, **28**(2):91–100.

Barrows, H.S. and Tamblyn, R. 1980 *Problem-Based Learning: An approach to medical education.* Springer, New York.

Bartlett, S.L. 1987 *When You Don't Know Where to Turn to: A self-diagnosing guide to counselling and therapy.* Contemporary Books, Chicago.

Baruth, L.G. 1987 *An Introduction to the Counselling Profession.* Prentice Hall, Englewood Cliffs, New Jersey.

Belkin, G.S. 1984 *Introduction to Counselling.* Brown, Dubuque, Iowa.

Benner, P. 1984 *From Novice to Expert.* Addison Wesley, California.

Benner, P. and Wrubel, J. 1989 *The Primacy of Caring: Stress and coping in health and illness.* Addison Wesley, California.

Berne, E. 1972 *What Do You Say After You Say Hello?* Corgi, London.

Bion, W.R. 1961 *Experiences in Groups.* Tavistock, London.

Black, K. 1983 *Short-Term Counselling: A humanistic approach for the helping professions.* Addison Wesley, London.

Bolger, A.W. (ed.) 1982 *Counselling in Britain: A reader.* Batsford Academic, London.

Bolton, E.B. 1980 A conceptual analysis of the mentoring relationship in the career development of women. *Adult Education*, **30**:195–207.

Bond, M. 1986 *Stress and Self-Awareness: A guide for nurses.* Heinemann, London.

Bond, M. and Kilty, J. 1986 *Practical Methods of Dealing with Stress*, 2nd edn. HPRP, University of Surrey, Guildford.

Boone, E.J., Shearon, R.W., White, E.E. *et al.* 1980 *Serving Personal and Community Needs through Adult Education.* Jossey Bass, San Francisco, California.

Boot, R. and Reynolds, M. 1983 Learning and Experience in Formal Education. Monograph. Department of Adult and Higher Education, University of Manchester.

Boud, D.J. (ed.) 1973 *Experiential Learning Techniques in Higher Education.* HPRP, University of Surrey, Guildford.

Boud, D.J. (ed.) 1981 *Developing Student Autonomy in Learning.* Kogan Page, London.

Boud, D.J. and Prosser, M.T. 1980 Sharing responsibility: staff–student cooperation in learning. *British Journal of Educational Technology*, **11**(1):24–35.

Boud, D.J., Keogh, R. and Walker, M. 1985 *Reflection: Turning experience into Learning.* Kogan Page, London.

Bowlby, J. 1975 *Separation.* Penguin, Harmondsworth.

Brandes, D. and Phillips, H. 1978 *The Gamester's Handbook.* Hutchinson, London.

Brandes, D. and Phillips, H. 1984 *The Gamester's Handbook*, vol. 2. Hutchinson, London.

Braswel, M. and Seay, T. 1984 *Approaches to Counselling and Psychotherapy.* Waverly, Prospect Heights, California.

Brown, A. 1979 *Groupwork.* Heinemann, London.

Brown, B.J. 1984 The dean as mentor. *Nursing Health Care*, **5**(2):88–91.

Brown, D. and Srebalus, D.J. 1988 *An Introduction to the Counselling Process.* Prentice Hall, Philadelphia.

Brown, L. 1986 The experience of care: patient perspectives. *Topics in Clinical Nursing*, **8**(2):56–62.

Brown, S.D. and Lent, R.W. (eds) 1984 *Handbook of Counselling Psychology.* John Wiley, Chichester.

Brunt, J.H. 1985 An exploration of the relationship between nurses' empathy and technology. *Nursing Administration Quarterly*, **9**(4):69–78.

Buerhaus, P. I. 1986 The economics of caring: challenges and new opportunities for nursing. *Topics in Clinical Nursing,* **8**(2):13–21.

Bugental, J.F.T. 1980 The far side of despair. *Journal of Humanistic Psychology,* **20**:49–68.

Bugental, E.K. and Bugental, J.F.T. 1984 Dispiritedness: a new perspective on a familiar state. *Journal of Humanistic Psychology,* **24**(1):49–67.

Burnard, P. 1988 The heart of the counselling relationship. *Senior Nurse,* **8**(12):17–18.

Burnard, P. 1988 Stress and relaxation in health visiting. *Health Visitor,* **61**(9):272.

Burnard, P. 1988 The spiritual needs of atheists and agnostics. *Professional Nurse,* **4**(3):130–2.

Burnard, P. 1989 Existentialism as a theoretical basis for counselling in psychiatric nursing. *Archives of Psychiatric Nursing,* **3**(3):142–7.

Burton, A. 1977 The mentoring dynamic in the therapuetic transformation. *American Journal of Psychoanalysis,* **37**:115–22.

Callner, D. and Ross, S. 1978 The assessment and training of assertiveness skills with drug addicts: a preliminary study. *International Journal of the Addictions,* **13**(2):227–30.

Campbell, A.V. 1981 *Rediscovering Pastoral Care.* Darton, Longman & Todd, London.

Carkuff, R.R. 1969 *Helping and Human Relations,* vol I, *Selection and Training.* Holt, Rinehart & Winston, New York.

Carson, B.V. 1989 *Spiritual Dimensions of Nursing Practice.* W.B. Saunders, Philadelphia.

Chapman, A.J. and Gale, A. 1982 *Psychology and People: A tutorial text.* British Psychological Society/Macmillan, London.

Chene, A. 1983 The concept of autonomy in adult education: a philosophical discusssion. *Adult Education Quarterly,* **32**(1):38–47.

Chickering, A.W. 1977 *Experience and Learning: An introduction to experiential learning.* Change Magazine Press, New Rochelle, New York.

Chickering, A.W. 1986 *Principles of Good Practice in Assessing Experiential Learning.* CAEL, Columbia, Maryland.

Chrousos, G.P., Loriaux, D.L. and Gold, P.W. 1988 *Mechanisms of Physical and Emotional Stress.* Plenum Press, New York.

Clark, M. 1978 Meeting the needs of the adult learner: using non-formal education for social action. *Convergence,* **XI**:34.

Clawson, J.G. 1985 Is mentoring necessary? *Training and Development Journal,* **39**(4):36–9.

Claxton, G. 1984 *Live and Learn: An introduction to the psychology of growth and change in everyday life.* Harper & Row, London.

Clift, J.C. and Imrie, B.W. 1981 *Assessing Students and Appraising Teaching.* Croom Helm, London.

Clutterbuck, D. 1985 *Everbody Needs a Mentor: How to further talent within an organisation.* Institute of Personnel Management, London.

Cohn, R. 1971 Living–learning encounters: the theme-centred interactional method. In G. Gottsgen, M. Gottsegen and L. Blank (eds) *Confrontation: Encounters in self and personal awareness.* Macmillan, London.

Coleman, J.S. 1982 Experiential learning and information assimilation: towards an appropriate mix. *Child and Youth Services,* **14**(3–4):12–20.

Collins, G.C. and Scott, P. 1979 Everyone who makes it has a mentor. *Harvard Business Review*, **56**:89–101.

Collins, N.W. 1983 *Professional Women and their Mentors*. Prentice Hall, Englewood Cliffs, New Jersey.

Conrad, D. and Hedin, D. 1982 The impact of experiential education on adolescent development. *Child and Youth Services*, **4**(3–4):57–76.

Conway, M.E. and Glass, L.K. 1978 Socialisation for survival in the academic world. *Nursing Outlook*, July, 324–429.

Corey, F. 1983 *I Never Knew I Had a Choice*, 2nd edn. Brooks Cole, Monterey, California.

Cormier, L.S. 1987 *The Professional Counsellor: A process guide to helping*. Prentice Hall, Englewood Cliffs, New Jersey.

Corsini, R. 1984 *Current Psychotherapies*, 3rd edn. Peacock, Itasca, Illinois.

Coser, R.L. 1962 *Life in the Ward*. Michigan State University, Michigan.

Cowan, J. and Garry, A. 1986 *Learning from Experience*. Further Education Unit, London.

Cox, T. 1978 *Stress*. Macmillan, London.

Cunningham, P.M. 1983 Helping students extract meaning from experience. In R.M. Smith (ed.) *Helping Adults Learn How To Learn: New directions for continuing education no. 19*. Jossey Bass, San Francisco.

Darling, L.W. 1986 What to do about toxic mentors. *Nurse Educator*, **11**(2):29–30.

Davis, C.M. 1981 Affective education for the health professions. *Physical Therapy*, **61**(11):1587–93.

Distance Learning Centre 1986 *Stress in Nursing: An open learning study pack*. Distance Learning Centre, South Bank Polytechnic, London.

Dixon, D.N. and Glover, J.A. 1984 *Counselling: A problem solving approach*. John Wiley, Chichester.

Douglas, T. 1976 *Groupwork Practice*. Tavistock, London.

Du Bois, E.E. 1982 Human resource development: expanding role. In C. Klevens (ed.) *Materials and Methods in Adult and Continuing Education*. Klevins Publications, Canoga Park, California.

Edelwich, J. and Brondsky, A. 1980 *Burnout: Stages of disillusionment in the helping professions*. Human Sciences Press, New York.

Edmunds, M. 1983 The nurse preceptor role. *Nurse Practitioner*, **8**(6):52–3.

Egan, G. 1977 *You and Me*. Brooks Cole, Monterey, California.

Egan, G. 1986 *Exercises in Helping Skills*, 3rd edn. Brooks Cole, Monterey, California.

Elbeck, M.A. 1986 Client perceptions of nursing practice. *Nursing Papers/ Perspectives in Nursing*, **18**(2):17–24.

Ellis, A. 1962 *Reason and Emotion in Psychotherapy*. Lyle, Stuart, New Jersey.

Ellis, R. (ed.) 1988 *Professional Competence and Quality Assurance in the Caring Professions*. Croom Helm, London.

Ellis, R. and Whittington, D. 1981 *A Guide to Social Skill Training*. Croom Helm, London.

Ernst, S. and Goodison, L. 1981 *In our own hands: A book of self help therapy*. Womens' Press, London.

Everly, G.S. and Rosenfeld, R. 1981 *The Nature and Treatment of the Stress Response: A practical guide for clinicians*. Plenum Press, New York.

Fabry, J. 1968 *The Pursuit of Meaning*. Beacon Press, Boston.

Fagan, M.M. and Walter, G. 1982 Mentoring among teachers. *Journal of Educational Research*, **76**(2):113–18.

Famighetti, R.A. 1981 Experiential learning: the close encounters of the institutional kind. *Gerontology and Geriatric Education*, **2**(2):129–32.

Fay, A. 1978 *Making Things Better by Making Them Worse*. Hawthorne, New York.

Fay, A. 1986 Clinical notes on paradoxical therapy. *Psychotherapy: Theory, Research and Practice*, **18**(1):14–22.

Feldenkrais, M. 1972 *Awareness Through Movement*. Harper & Row, New York.

Ferruci, P. 1982 *What We May Be*. Turnstone Press, Wellingborough.

Fiedler, F.E. 1950 The concept of an ideal therapeutic relationship. *Journal of Consulting Psychology*, **14**:239–45.

Fisher, J. 1981 A continuing education workshop on human relations. *Nursing Papers*, **13**(3):27–36.

Fisher, S. and Reason, J. 1988 *Handbook of Life Stress: Cognition and health*. John Wiley, Chichester.

Foggo-Pays, E. 1983 *An Introductory Guide to Counselling*. Ravenswood, Beckenham.

Fontana, D. 1989 *Managing Stress*. British Psychological Society/Routledge, London.

Fordham, F. 1966 *An Introduction to Jung's Psychology*. Penguin, Harmondsworth.

Fox, F.E. 1983 The spiritual core of experiential education. *Journal of Experiential Education*, **16**(1):3–6.

Frankl, V.E. 1959 *Man's Search for Meaning*. Beacon Press, New York.

Frankl, V.E. 1969 *The Will to Meaning*. World Publishing, New York.

Frankl, V.E. 1975 Paradoxical intention and dereflection: a logotherapuetic technique. *Psychotherapy: Theory, Research and Practice*, **12**(3):226–37.

Frankl, V.E. 1975 *The Unconcious God*. Simon & Schuster, New York.

Frankl, V.E. 1978 *The Unheard Cry for Meaning*. Simon & Schuster, New York.

Freudenberger, H. and Richelson, G. 1974 *Burnout: How to beat the high cost of success*. Bantam Books, New York.

Fromm, E. 1941 *Escape from Freedom*. Avon, New York.

Gaut, D.A. 1983 Development of a theoretically adequate description of caring. *Western Journal of Nursing Research*, **5**(4):313–23.

Geller, L. 1985 Another look at self-actualisation. *Journal of Humanistic Psychology*, **24**(2):93–106.

Gendlin, E.T. and Beebe, J. 1968 An experiential approach to group therapy. *Journal of Research and Developments in Education*, **1**:19–29.

George, P. and Kummerow, J. 1981 Mentoring for career women. *Training*, **18**(2):44–9.

Gibson, R.L. and Mitchell, M.H. 1986 *Introduction to Counselling and Guidance*. Collier Macmillan, London.

Gilfoyle, E.M. 1980 Caring: a philosophy for practice. *American Journal of Occupational Therapy*, **34**(8):517–21.

Gladstein, G.A. 1983 Understanding empathy: integrating counselling, developmental and social psychology perspectives. *Journal of Counselling Psychology*, **30**(4):467–82.

Goffman, E. 1968 *Asylums: Essays on the social situation of mental patients and other inmates*. Penguin, Harmondsworth.

Golan, N. 1981 *Passing Through Transitions: A guide for practitioners*. Free Press, New York.

Goldberg, L. and Beznitz, S. 1982 *Handbook of Stress: Theoretical and Clinical Aspects.* Macmillan, New York.

Guggenbühl-Craig, A. 1971 *Power in the Helping Professions.* Spring, University of Dallas, Irving, Texas.

Haas, J. and Shaggir, W. 1982 Ritual evaluation of competence: the hidden curriculum of professionalization in an innovative medical school program. *Work and Occupation,* **2**:131–54.

Halmos, P. 1965 *The Faith of the Counsellors.* Constable, London.

Hamilton, M.S. 1981 Mentorhood: a key to nursing leadership. *Nursing Leadership,* **4**(1):4–13.

Hamrick, M. and Stone, C. 1979 Promoting experiential learning. *Health Education,* **10**(4):38–41.

Hanks, L., Belliston, L. and Edwards, D. 1977 *Design Yourself.* Kaufman, Los Altos, California.

Hanson, J. 1986 *The Joy of Stress.* Pan, London.

Harris, T. 1969 *I'm O.K., You're O.K.* Harper & Row, London.

Health Education Authority, High Stress Occupation Working Party 1988. *Stress in the Public Sector: Nurses, police, social workers and teachers.* Health Education Authority.

Heap, K. 1979 *Process and Action in Work with Groups.* Pergamon Press, Oxford.

Hendricks, G. and Fadiman, J. (eds) 1976 *Transpersonal Education: a curriculum for feeling and being.* Prentice Hall, Englewood Cliffs, New Jersey.

Henry, C. and Tuxill, A.C. 1987 Persons and humans. *Journal of Advanced Nursing,* **12**:383–8.

Herinck, R. (ed.) 1980 *The Psychotherapy Handbook.* New American Library, New York.

Heron, J. 1973 *Experience and Method.* HPRP, University of Surrey, Guildford, Surrey.

Heron, J. 1974 *The Concept of a Peer Learning Community.* HPRP, University of Surrey, Guildford.

Heron, J. 1978 *Co-Counselling Teacher's Manual.* HPRP, University of Surrey, Guildford, Surrey.

Heron, J. 1981 *Experiential Research: A New Paradigm.* HPRP, University of Surrey, Guildford.

Heron, J. 1989 *A Handbook of Facilitator Style.* Kogan Page, London.

Hewitt, J. 1977 *Meditation.* Hodder & Stoughton, Sevenoaks, Kent.

Hingley, P. and Cooper, C.L. 1986 *Stress and the Nurse Manager.* John Wiley, Chichester.

Holt, R. 1982 An alternative to mentorship. *Adult Education,* **55**(2):152–6.

Hurding, R.F. 1985 *Roots and Shoots: A guide to counselling and psychotherapy.* Hodder & Stoughton, London.

Hutchins, D.E. 1987 *Helping Relationships and Strategies.* Brooks Cole, Monterey, California.

Ivey, A.E. 1987 *Counselling and Psychotherapy: Skills, theories and practice.* Prentice Hall, London.

Jackins, H. 1965 *The Human Side of Human Beings.* Rational Island Publishers, Seattle, Washington.

Jackins, H. 1970 *Fundamentals of Co-Counselling Manual.* Rational Island Publishers, Seattle, Washington.

Jacobson, S.F. 1983 Stresses and coping strategies of neonatal intensive care unit nurses, research in nursing and health. *Practitioner* **6**(226):1580–2.

James, M. and Jongeward, D. 1971 *Born to Win: Transactional analysis with Gestalt experiments.* Addison Wesley, Reading, Massachusetts.

Jarvis, P. 1987 *Adult Learning in the Social Context.* Croom Helm, London.

Jarvis, P. 1987 Meaningful and meaningless experience: towards an understanding of learning from life. *Adult Education Quarterly,* **37**:3.

Jenkins, E. 1987 *Facilitating Self Awareness: A learning package combining group work with computer assisted learning.* Croom Helm, London.

Johnson, J.A., Cheek, J.M. and Smither, R. 1983 The structure of empathy. *Journal of Personality and Social Psychology,* **45**:1299–312.

Jung, C.G. 1976 *Modern Man in Search of a Soul.* Routledge & Kegan Paul, London.

Jung, C.G. 1978 In A. Storr (ed.) *Selected Writings.* Fontana, London.

Kahn, R.L. and Cannell, C.F. 1957 *The Dynamics of Interviewing.* John Wiley, New York.

Kanter, R.M. 1979 *Men and Women of the Corporation.* Basic Books, New York.

Kast, F.E. and Rosenzweig, J.E. 1978 *Organisation and Management: A systems and contingency approach,* 2nd edn. McGraw-Hill, New York.

Kennedy, E. 1979 *On Becoming a Counsellor.* Gill and Macmillan, London.

Kleinman, A. 1988 *The Illness Narratives: Suffering, healing and the human condition.* Basic Books, New York.

Klopf, G.J. and Harrison, J. 1981 Moving up the career ladder: the case for mentors. *Principal,* **61**(1):41–3.

Knowles, M.S. 1975 *Self-Directed Learning: A guide for learners and teachers.* Cambridge, New York.

Knox, A.B. (ed.) 1980 *Teaching Adults Effectively.* Jossey Bass, San Francisco, California.

Koberg, D. and Bagnal, J. 1981 *The Revised All New Universal Traveler: A soft-systems guide to creativity, problem-solving and the process of reaching goals.* Kaufmann, Los Altos, California.

Kolb, D.A., Rubin, I.M. and McIntyre, J.M. 1984 *Organizational Psychology: An experiential approach to organizational behaviour.* Prentice Hall, Englewood Cliffs, New Jersey.

Kottler, J.A. and Brown, R.W. 1985 *Introduction to Therapeutic Counselling.* Brooks Cole, Monterey, California.

Krebs, D.L. and Miller, D.T. 1985 Altruism and aggression. In G. Lindzey and E. Aronson (eds) *Handbook of Social Psychology,* vol. 2, 3rd edn. Random House, New York.

La Monica, E.L. 1981 Construct validity of an empathy instrument. *Research in Nursing and Health,* **4**:389–400.

La Monica, E.L. 1983 The nurse as helper: today and tomorrow. In N.L. Chaska (ed.) *The Nursing Profession: A time to speak.* McGraw-Hill, Toronto.

La Monica, E.L., Wolf, R.M., Madea, A.R. and Oberst, M.T. 1987 *Empathy and Nursing Outcomes: Scholarly inquiry for nursing practice,* **1**:197–213.

Lachman, V.D. 1983 *Stress Management: A manual for nurses.* Grune & Stratton, Orlando, Florida.

Lazarus, R.S. and Folkman, S. 1984 *Stress, Appraising and Coping.* Springer, New York.

Leech, K. 1986 *Spirituality and Pastoral Care.* Sheldon Press, London.

Leggieri, J. 1986 Pastoral care in the hospital: uniqueness and contribution. *Topics in Clinical Nursing,* **8**(2):47–55.

Leininger, M.M. 1988 *Care: Discovery and uses in clinical and community nursing*. Wayne State University Press, Detroit.

Lieberman, M.A. 1978 Self-help groups: problems of measuring outcomes. *Small Group Behaviour*, **9**:221–41.

Lomas, P. 1973 *True and False Experience*. Allen Lane, London.

Lowen, A. 1967 *Betrayal of the Body*. Macmillan, New York.

Lowen, A and Lowen, L. 1977 *The Way to Vibrant Health: A manual of bioenergetic exercises*. Harper & Row, New York.

Luft, J. 1969 *Of Human Interaction: The Johari model*. Mayfield, Palo Alto, California.

Lundberg, R. 1985 What kind of good is a kind and caring heart? *Journal of Value Inquiry*, **19**:119–31.

McIntee, J. and Firth, H. 1984 How to beat the burnout. *Health and Social Services Journal*, 9 February, 166–8.

Madders, J. 1980 *Stress and Relaxation*. Martin Dunitz, London.

Marshall, E.K. and Kurtz, P.D. (eds) 1982 *Interpersonal Helping Skills: A guide to training methods, programs and resources*. Jossey Bass, San Francisco, California.

Maslach, C. 1981 *Burnout: The cost of caring*. Prentice Hall, Englewood Cliffs, New Jersey.

May, C. 1990 Research on nurse–patient relationships: problems of theory, problems of practice. *Journal of Advanced Nursing*, **15**:307–15.

Mayeroff, M. 1965 On caring. *International Philosophy Quarterly*, **5**:462–74.

Meichenbaum, D. 1983 *Coping With Stress*. Century Publishing, London.

Meichenbaum, D. and Jaremko, M.E. 1983 *Stress Reduction and Prevention*. Plenum Press, New York.

Merriam, S. 1984 Mentors and protégés: a critical review of the literature. *Adult Education Quarterly*, **33**(3):161–73.

Miller, A. 1985 Cognitive styles and environmental problem solving. *International Journal of Environmental Studies*, **26**:21–31.

Morse, J.M. 1991 Negotiating commitment and involvement in the nurse–patient relationship. *Journal of Advanced Nursing*, **16**:455–68.

Morsund, J. 1985 *The Process of Counselling and Therapy*. Prentice Hall, Englewood Cliffs, New Jersey.

Mouton, J.S. and Blake, R.R. 1984 *Synergogy: A new strategy for education, training and development*. Jossey Bass, San Francisco, California.

Murgatroyd, S. 1986 *Counselling and Helping*. British Psychological Society/Methuen, London.

Murgatroyd, S. and Woolfe, R. 1982 *Coping with Crisis – Understanding and Helping Persons in Need*. Harper & Row, London.

Nadler, L. (ed.) 1984 *The Handbook of Human Resource Development*. John Wiley, New York.

Naranjo, C. and Ornstein, R.E. 1971 *On the Psychology of Meditation*. Allen & Unwin, London.

Nelson-Jones, R. 1983 *Practical Counselling Skills: A psychological skills approach for the helping professions and for voluntary counsellors*. Holt, Rinehart & Winston, London.

Nelson-Jones, R. 1984 *Personal Responsibility: Counselling and therapy: An integrative approach*. Harper & Row, London.

Nelson-Jones, R. 1988 *Practical Counselling and Helping Skills: Helping clients to help themselves*. Cassell, London.

Nichols, K.A. 1993 *Psychological Care in Physical Illness*. Chapman & Hall, London.

Noddings, N. 1981 Caring. *Journal of Curriculum Theorising*, **3**(2):139–48.

Ohlsen, A.M., Horne, A.M. and Lawe, C.F. 1988 *Group Counselling*. Holt, Rinehart & Winston, New York.

Open University Coping With Crisis Group 1987 *Running Workshops: A guide for trainers in the helping professions*. Croom Helm, London.

Ornstein, R.E. 1975 *The Psychology of Consciousness*. Penguin, Harmondsworth.

Patton, M.Q. 1982 *Practical Evaluation*. Sage, Beverly Hills, California.

Payne, R. and Firth-Cozens, J. 1987 *Stress in Health Professionals*. John Wiley, Chichester.

Pedlar, M. (ed.) 1983 *Action Learning in Practice*. Gower, London.

Peplau, H.E. 1988 *Interpersonal Relations in Nursing*. Macmillan, London.

Perls, F., Hefferline, R.F. and Goodman, P. 1951 *Gestalt Therapy: Excitement and growth in the human personality*. Penguin, Harmondsworth.

Phillip-Jones, L. 1982 *Mentors and Protégés*. Arbour House, New York.

Phillip-Jones, L. 1983 Establishing a formalised mentoring programme. *Training and Development Journal*, February, 38–42.

Polyani, M. 1958 *Personal Knowledge*. University of Chicago Press, Chicago.

Porrit, L. 1990 *Interaction Strategies: An introduction for health professionals*, 2nd edn. Churchill Livingstone, Edinburgh.

Procter, B. 1978 *Counselling Shop: An introduction to the theories and techniques of ten approaches to counselling*. Deutsch, London.

Rawlings, M.E. and Rawlings, L. 1983 Mentoring and networking for helping professionals. *Personnel and Guidance Journal*, **62**(2):116–18.

Reddy, M. 1987 *The Manager's Guide to Counselling at Work*. Methuen, London.

Rempusheski, V.F., Chamberalin, S.L., Picard, H.B., Ruzanski, J. and Collier, M. 1988 Expected and received care: patient perceptions. *Nursing Administration Quarterly*, **12**(3):42–50.

Revans, R. 1980 *Action Learning*. Blond & Briggs, London.

Riebel, L. 1984 A homeopathic model of psychotherapy. *Journal of Humanistic Psychology*, **24**(1):9–48.

Riemen, D.J. 1986 Non-caring and caring in the clinical setting: patients' descriptions. *Topics in Clinical Nursing*, **8**(2):30–6.

Ringuette, E.L. 1983 A note on experiential learning in professional training. *Journal of Clinical Psychology*, **39**(2):302–4.

Robinson, L. 1968 *Psychological Aspects of the Care of Hospitalised Patients*. F.A. Davis, Philadelphia.

Roche, G.R. 1979 Much ado about mentors. *Harvard Business Review*, **56**:14–28.

Rogers, C.R. and Stevens, B. 1967 *Person to Person: The problem of being human*. Real People Press, Lafayette, California.

Rowan, J. 1986 Holistic listening. *Journal of Humanistic Psychology*, **26**(1):83–102.

Rushton, J.P. and Sorrentino, R.M. 1981 Altruism and helping behaviour: an historical perspective. In J.P. Rushton and R.M. Sorrentino (eds) *Altruism and Helping Behaviour: Social, personality and developmental perspectives*. Lawrence Erlbaum, Hillsdale, New Jersey.

Sabini, J. and Silver, M. 1985 On the captivity of the will: sympathy, caring and a moral sense of the human. *Journal for the Theory of Social Behaviour*, **15**(1):23–37.

Scheler, M. 1954 *The Nature of Sympathy*, 5th edn (P. Heath trans.). Routledge & Kegan Paul, London.

Schmidt, J.A. and Wolfe, J.S. 1980 The mentor partnership: discovery of professionalism. *NASPA Journal*, **17**:45–51.

Schon, D.A. 1983 *The Reflective Practitioner: How professionals think in action*. Basic Books, New York.

Schorr, T.M. 1978 The lost art of mentoring. *American Journal of Nursing*, **78**:1873.

Schulman, D. 1982 *Intervention in Human Services: A guide to skills and knowledge*, 3rd edn. C.V. Mosby, St Louis, Missouri.

Shapiro, E.C., Haseltime, F. and Rowe, M. 1978 Moving up: role models, mentors and the patron system. *Sloan Management Review*, **19**:51–8.

Shropshire, C.O. 1981 Group experiential learning in adult education. *Journal of Continuing Education in Nursing*, **12**:(6)5–9.

Simon, S.B., Howe, L.W. and Kirschenbaum, H. 1978 *Values Clarification*, rev. edn. A and W Visual Library, New York.

Smith, P. 1992 *The Emotional Labour of Nursing. Its Impact on Interpersonal Relations, Management and the Educational Environment in Nursing*. Macmillan, London.

Smith, S. 1986 *Communications in Nursing: Communicating assertively and responsibly in nursing*. McGraw-Hill, Toronto.

Speizer, J.J. 1981 Role models, mentors and sponsors: the elusive concept. *Signs*, **6**:692–712.

Stevenson, L. 1987 *Seven Theories of Human Nature*, 2nd edn. Oxford University Press, Oxford.

Taylor, S. 1986 Mentors: who are they and what are they doing? *Thrust For Educational Leadership*, **15**(7):39–41.

Tillich, P. 1952 *The Courage to Be*. Yale University Press, New Haven, Connecticut.

Toi, M. and Batson, C.D. 1982 More evidence that empathy is a source of altruistic motivation. *Journal of Personality and Social Psychology*, **43**(2):281–92.

Tough, A.M. 1982 *Intentional Changes: A fresh approach to helping people change*. Cambridge Books, New York.

Tuckman, B.W. 1965 Developmental sequences in small groups. *Psychological Bulletin*, **63**:384–99.

Van den Berg, J.H. 1972 *The Psychology of the Sickbed*. Humanities Press, New York.

Vickers, G. 1983 *Human Systems are Different*. Harper & Row, London.

Wallace, W.A. 1986 *Theories of Counselling and Psychotherapy: A basic issues approach*. Allyn & Bacon, Boston.

Wallis, R. 1984 *Elementary Forms of the New Religious Life*. Routledge & Kegan Paul, London.

Walters, G.A. and Marks, S.E. 1981 *Experiential Learning and Change: Theory, design and practice*. John Wiley, New York.

Weatley, D. 1981 *Stress and the Heart: Interactions of the cardiovascular system, behaviour states and psychotropic drugs*. Raven Press, New York.

Wheeler, D.D. and Janis, I.L. 1980 *A Practical Guide for Making Decisions*. Free Press, New York.

Whitaker, D.S. 1985 *Using Groups To Help People*. Tavistock/Routledge, London.

Wlodkowski, R.J. 1985 *Enhancing Adult Motivation to Learn*. Jossey Bass, San Francisco, California.

Index